PREDATORS

PREDATORS

Pedophiles, Rapists, and Other Sex Offenders

Who They Are,

How They Operate,

and How We Can Protect

Ourselves and Our Children

ANNA C. SALTER, PH.D.

BASIC BOOKS

A Member of the Perseus Books Group
New York

Hardback edition first published in 2003 by Basic Books,
A Member of the Perseus Books Group
Paperback edition first published in 2004 by Basic Books.

Books published by Basic Books are available at special discounts for bulk purchases
in the United States by corporations, institutions, and other organizations. For more
information, please contact the Special Markets Department at the Perseus Books
Group, 11 Cambridge Center, Cambridge MA 02142, or call (617) 252-5298,
(800) 255-1514 or e-mail special.markets@perseusbooks.com.

Designed by Brent Wilcox

Library of Congress has catalogued the hardcover edition as follows:
Salter, Anna C.
    Predators : pedophiles, rapists, and other sex offenders : who they are, how they
operate, and how we can protect ourselves and our children / Anna C. Salter
        p.   cm.
    Includes bibliographical references and index.
    ISBN 0-465-07172-4 (hc)
    1. Sex offenders.   2. Sex offenders—Psychology.   3. Sexual deviation.
I. Title.
ISBN-13 978-0-465-07173-9
ISBN-10 0-465-07173-2 (pbk)

HQ71 .S28   2003
364.15'3—dc21
                                                                    2002015846

10 9

As always,

For BLAKE and JAZZY

"Because joy is the only thing that slows the clock"

—JOHN MACDONALD

CONTENTS

FOREWORD

I'm beginning this Foreword as I will close it: Thank you, Anna Salter, for casting your authoritative light on sexual abuse while most people find it easier to look away or even deny that it exists. It is easier for most parents to wring their hands about the unknown molester who might wander into the neighborhood than to accept that someone who they invited into the house is sexually abusing their child—even though the majority of sexual abuse is committed by someone the family knows.

Hard as it is to accept the idea that a well-liked neighbor or family friend might be sexually abusing a child, imagine the idea that it's someone in your own family. It's easy to replace that unwelcome thought with a warmer one like, "Not in *this* family."

And yet one in three girls and one in six boys will have sexual contact with an adult, so it must be occurring in someone's family. Wherever sexual abuse occurs, there are unwitting parents or caregivers witnessing the performance that precedes the crime, choosing not to see clearly as predators persuade children to trust them. Naïve parents are often unconscious co-conspirators in cases of sexual abuse, designing theories to explain the onset of a child's sleep disturbances or eating problems or sudden fear of that same adult she liked so much just a week ago.

If a discussion requires exploration of harsh truths some parents will try to wriggle away: "Talking about those things, you just bring them on," or "Yes, I know all about that stuff; can we please change to a happier subject?" Under pressure, though, they will ultimately acknowledge the risks, realizing that appearing to know is often the best defense against unwanted knowledge. These parents are not stupid—to the contrary, there is brilliance in the creative ways that they exclude their children from the dis-

cussion. "You're so right," they say: "Sexual abuse is an enormous problem, particularly for young teens. Thank God mine aren't there yet."

*No, sorry, says reality, the most common age at which sexual abuse be-
gins is three.*

"Well, sure, if you have homosexuals around small children, there's a
risk."

*No, sorry, says reality, most sexual abuse is committed by heterosexual
males.*

"Yeah, but that kind of pervert isn't living in our neighborhood."

*Sorry, says reality, but that kind of pervert is living in your neighbor-
hood. The Department of Justice estimates that on average, there is one
child molester per square mile in the United States.*

"Well, at least the police know who these people are."

*Not likely, says reality, since the average child molester victimizes be-
tween 50 and 150 children before he is ever arrested (and many more after
he is arrested).*

When all defenses against reality are taken away, some parents
switch to resignation, literally resigning from responsibility: "Well,
there's nothing you can do about it anyway." This misplaced fatalism
actually becomes fatal for some children.

Another common refrain uttered by deniers of the dangers of sexual
abuse is: "Well, kids are resilient. When bad things happen, they
bounce back."

*Absolutely not, says reality. Children do not bounce back. They adjust,
they conceal, they repress, and sometimes they accept and move on, but
they don't bounce back.*

If I seem hard on denial, I have my reasons, reasons that make me
grateful the pages of *Predators* contain an antidote to denial: well-
researched, clearly presented information. We learn from Anna Salter
that the sexual offender is also in denial, that he is a criminal who
chooses to stay on the road he is on even when it's clear where it will
carry him. Salter has interviewed enough sexual offenders to learn the
most alarming truth: Many feel entitled to every predatory prize they
can win and simply do not care about the cost to others. They are, in
short, cruel.

And for virtually every cruelty done to a child, there is an audience of deniers that sees the signals and quickly closes their eyes.

The solution to sexual violence in America is not more laws, more guns, more police, or more prisons. *The solution to sexual violence is acceptance of reality.*

One of the starkest realities is that sexual predators are stunningly effective at gaining control over their victims.

There are two basic predatory types, the power-predator and the persuasion-predator. The power-predator charges like a bear, unmistakably committing to his attack. Because of this, he cannot easily retreat and say there was merely a misunderstanding. Accordingly, he strikes only when he feels certain he'll prevail.

The far more common offender is a persuasion-predator. This type of criminal looks for a vulnerable victim, someone who will allow him to be in control. Like a shark circling potential prey, the persuasion-predator approaches slowly and watches to see how people react to his advances. He begins a dialogue and with each favorable response he elicits, he circles closer. He makes a small initial investment, a low-risk strategy that allows him to test the waters and move on with nobody the wiser if things don't go well. He is a coward, a crafty one, but a coward nonetheless.

A predator's selection of victims can be as complex and inexplicable as sexual attraction is for adults, with one important distinction: For most pedophiles, vulnerability is, all by itself, stimulating. Just as with animals, human predators must separate their targets from the flock. Taking children from parents is rarely done with force; kids are not stolen at gunpoint. They are taken through a form of seduction, one that aims not at passion, but at trust—yours or your child's. Misplaced trust is the predator's most powerful resource, and we can decide whether or not to give it to him.

Misplaced trust can have terrible consequences. In addition to what we usually think of as molestation, children are victims of rape more often than most of us have ever imagined. The Bureau of Justice Statistics reports that fully 15% of rape victims are younger than twelve.

A mother named Carla told me of taking her six-year-old daughter to the small fenced playground at their local park. Most of the children there were accompanied by a parent, a few by babysitters or nannies, one by a grandparent. After a short while, Carla had intuitively connected each child to his or her guardian. In one case, it was because they resembled each other; in another, she saw a child run up and say something to an adult. She heard one man call out some encouragement to a boy who was hesitating at the top of a slide. Soon enough, Carla had accounted for every adult in the playground but one man, one man she didn't like.

He was sitting on a bench watching the children play, but he was not focused on any particular child. He had nothing with him, while most of the other adults had something they were keeping an eye on: a doll, a toy, a stroller with a blanket on the seat. When Carla saw the man leave the playground alone, she thought, *I don't trust him. What was he doing here anyway? Glad he's gone. I'll watch for him in the future. He seemed like a child molester.*

Seemed like a child molester? On the basis of what? One might call this an outrageous and unearned condemnation, a discrimination so intolerant that it would be illegal in any other context. When the man came back to the playground a few minutes later and Carla saw his son run up and hug him (she'd wrongly connected that boy to another adult), she quickly forgave her own prejudice. After all, she told me later, "I was just protecting my child."

I asked if she felt bad for having falsely accused the man in her mind. *Nope.* Did the experience make her reluctant to judge people so quickly in the future? *Nope.* Even though he turned out to be just another parent, did she regret her suspiciousness? *Nope.*

After praising her self-confidence, I pointed out, "To effectively protect your daughter, you'd need to be just as willing to entertain suspicions about people you know."

"That's not quite as easy," Carla responded, "because then I'd feel terribly guilty."

This kind of misplaced guilt is problematic because a child is far more vulnerable to someone the family knows than to a stranger. And Carla, like any parent, is far more resistant to suspecting someone she knows. The people we willingly suspect are inherently less dangerous than those we refuse to suspect. We tend to suppress objectionable thoughts about our friends, but the only way to really banish a thought is to fully consider it. In fact, we are treating our friends with greater respect and our children with greater love when we are willing to entertain, and hopefully dismiss, the possibility that the people close to us may be capable of sexual abuse.

My point is not that you ought to distrust a man or teenage boy merely because he has access to your children, but that you must be willing to trust your intuition when you do feel suspicion. Above all, I encourage parents to make careful, slow choices about the people they include in their children's lives—and fast choices about the people they exclude. It is a feature of our species that some of the adult males molest children. Expecting those particular males to look glaringly different from all others has proved to be an ineffective strategy for preventing sexual abuse. Popular, but ineffective.

When it comes to the safety of children, I've concluded that the primary difference between parents and experts is that parents say "I guess" more often—as in "I guess these molesters hang around places frequented by kids." And parents end their statements with question marks: "Kids are less vulnerable in pairs, right?" Since the information remains roughly the same no matter who offers it, I show whenever possible that what people think the answer might be is, in fact, exactly what it usually turns out to be. I recall a mother who asked me how to identify the signs of child abuse.

I responded with a question: "What do you think the signs are?"

"I don't know."

"If you did know the answer, what would it be?" (This almost always stimulates an answer from the very person who just said I don't know.)

"Well, I guess sleep problems. Maybe the child's behavior changes—but other than that, I don't know."

"You mean that other than knowing, you don't know?"

"I don't know."

"If you did know, what other signs might there be?"

"Acting sort of sexual with other kids? Drawing pictures about sex? Doing sexual things? I don't know."

Right on all points, of course. If you add hyperactivity, fear of being alone with certain adults, unusual or exaggerated interest in people's bodies, wearing excessive amounts of clothing, you'd have several of the most common behavioral signs.

Sometimes a child's body will clearly say what's happened, and those clues are far harder to miss. This list tells the story so starkly that it hurts your heart to read it:

- Stomach pains and digestive problems
- Difficulty walking or sitting
- Torn, stained, or bloody underwear
- Blood in urine or stool
- Unexplained genital contusions
- Sexually transmitted diseases
- Pregnancy

Lists like that are part of what makes this a topic nobody really wants to think about. Accordingly, too few parents do think about it, while too many predators are perfecting their skills.

In addition to the denial of some parents, predators are served by several evolving social factors. More mothers are working, so more children are spending their days in childcare facilities. Divorce is on the rise, and the increasing number of remarriages means more sexual abuse by stepfathers in the home. Research has shown that boyfriends or stepfathers are much more likely to abuse their partner's child that the child's biological father. Sexual crimes against children also increase as victims of abuse grow up to become abusers themselves. Finally, since most sexual predators molest many children, the number of victims is increasing exponentially.

Predators gives parents and educators the best kind of defense against sexual offenders: wisdom. On behalf of all the children and adults who will, because of this book, never become victims at all, I would like to say: Thank you Anna Salter.

—*Gavin de Becker*

ACKNOWLEDGMENTS

First there is the writing and the people who helped with it. I was lucky on this book to have several professionals involved who do an exceptional job. I want to thank my editor, Jo Ann Miller of Basic Books, whose feedback was always thoughtful and always beneficial. I am always grateful to my agent, Helen Rees, a consummate professional, who has guided me since my first mystery. Finally, I want to thank William Patrick, who edited the book privately, for his carefully considered comments and suggestions.

In addition, as with all my books, I seek out specialists in the area to read and critique it for errors. For this book, the following experts were particularly helpful: Gary McCaughtry, the Warden of Waupan Correctional Institution in Waupan, Wisconsin; Margaret Alexander, Clinical Director of the Sex Offender Treatment Program at Oshkosh Correctional Institute in Oshkosh, Wisconsin; Suzanne Schmitt, Section Chief of the Program Planning and Evaluation, Department of Corrections, Madison, Wisconsin; Steve and Cory Jensen, sex offender treatment providers in Portland, Oregon; Lynne Henderson, Professor of Law at the Boyd School of Law, University of Nevada, Las Vegas; and Stephanie Dallam, research associate for the Leadership Council for Mental Health, Justice and the Media. The latter is an excellent organization, and I would recommend that anyone who wants accurate information about sexual abuse try their website at www.Leadershipcouncil.org.

Finally, there were friends outside the field who read the book for sense and readability. My mentor, Regina Yando, has read and critiqued all my books, and they are stronger for it. Merija Eisen, a friend and neighbor, showed an unusual gift for editing. My friend Renee Sandler read the final draft with an Alaskan eagle eye.

Finally, there are people I want to thank just because they make the world a little safer: Ken Pope, who more than anyone else has brought the field of sexual abuse experts together; Andrew Vachss for his tireless support of children; Steve and Cory Jensen and Roger and Florence Wolfe because they run treatment programs that work; Dennis Doren for his informed and thoughtful approach to evaluating sex offenders; Eric Holden because he's shown just how good a polygrapher can be; and Tony Streveler, my boss at the Wisconsin Department of Corrections, because he is a visionary and a man of warmth and humor; he keeps my cynicism within the bounds of sanity. Finally, I want to thank the late Fay Honey Knopp, who got us all started in the first place. Honey, wherever you are, this one's for you.

For anyone who wants to contact me, my website is http://www.AnnaSalter.com.

Introduction

As a young therapist in the late 1970s, I took my Ph.D. in psychology to a small town in New England, expecting to have a general practice and to live the country life. I envisioned child clients with problems with attention and behavior, some consulting to local schools, a garden, perhaps a horse.

But it seemed two out of three children I saw in the small mental health center where I worked were sexually or physically abused or both. That struck me as very odd indeed. At the time, official estimates suggested incest affected one child in a million. My small New England town had 15,000 people in it, yet it had a stunning number of incest cases, not to mention out-of-home sexual abuse, rape, physical abuse, neglect, and domestic violence.

One year, driven by a desperate passion for a thoroughbred with legs of spun glass and a close relationship with the local vet, I worked mental health emergency, covering an entire county, every third night. It was a crushing schedule, and I did it to support the horse, but what I learned was priceless. Working emergency—especially for so many nights—made the violence stark and present in an immediate, visceral way not found in more distant, weekly therapy sessions. I learned to say to callers who complained that their husbands beat them, "Is he beating you now?" Often he was, and they were calling in the hope that I could somehow magically stop it over the phone without their having to leave him. At best, the beating just got postponed.

Over time I developed the fantasy that my small town in New England was similar to the square mile in Mexico where all the monarch butterflies go. It must be, I thought, the center of violence in the known universe. It had to be, if the official estimates of violence were right, because there wasn't supposed to be that much violence anywhere, certainly not in small towns in the United States. In the two years I spent at Tufts getting a Masters degree in Child Study and the five years I spent at Harvard getting a Ph.D. in Psychology and Public Practice, there was virtually nothing on child sexual and physical abuse in any course I took. I had one lecture on the victims of child abuse, but not a single lecture anywhere on offenders. Ironically, many of the lectures were on maladies so rare I've yet to see them in twenty years of practice.

In the years since, I've met many clinicians in different towns and cities all over the United States with the same fantasy that their own towns or cities were the center of violence in the universe. After a lecture on sexual abuse, a member of the audience will speak with me. "Do you think there's more sexual abuse in small towns?" she will say to me, puzzled. "We're seeing so much of it."

A few minutes later, someone else will come up, "Do you think there's more in cities?" he will ask. "I just wonder because we get so many cases." This nation's dirty little secret—only now getting a modicum of attention because of the crisis of pedophilic priests in the Catholic church—is the number of domestic violence, rape, and child molestation cases that are never reported to police.

At the time, back in the late 1970s, some naïve part of me thought something was being done about sexual and violent offenders, at least once the abuse was reported. I just assumed—when the child reported, when the reports were specific and graphic, in cases where the mother believed the child and the authorities were informed—that the perpetrator was being apprehended, tried, convicted. I believed the same about rape. Then the day came when a five-year-old named the same offender that another five-year-old had several years before. "Wait a minute," I thought. "Is he still out there? Didn't somebody do something about him?" No one had.

What I didn't grasp at the time was that no one knew what to do. In a child sexual abuse case, courts were not likely to take the word of a four-year-old over an elder in the church, much less the pastor in the church. Offenders were rarely stupid. They weren't slow to realize that if they restricted themselves to preschoolers, then their chances of a conviction were virtually zero. The few who were convicted served little time, and in any case, they were all released eventually, usually without the benefit of any kind of specialized treatment. Most rapes I heard about were never reported at all.

"Volunteer" clients, offenders who weren't ordered into therapy by a judge, rarely stuck with therapy. There was almost always someone behind them, I discovered—a spouse, a neighbor, someone who promised not to report the abuse if he[1] would just "get help." He would get help—for the few weeks it took for the neighbors or spouses to relax their guard. Then he would disappear from therapy, usually with high praise for my services. "Doc," he'd say, "this is the best thing that ever happened to me. I can't tell you how much I've learned. Well, I guess I won't be doing that anymore. I don't think I need any more therapy. Thank you very much. You're the greatest."

I would realize, with heart-stopping dismay, that I had no release to tell the neighbors or spouses that he had even dropped out of therapy—not in those early days. The spouses or neighbors would go on their way, secure in the knowledge that the offender was "getting help." Every time I opened the newspaper I feared I would see one of my former clients in the headlines.

Without doing something about the perpetrator, I felt therapy for victims was only a stopgap measure. Victims were the result, not the cause, of the problem. Providing services to victims should be a priority, but it wouldn't do much to reduce the chances that another child or adult was placed in harm's way.

But what could be done about offenders? All offenders are likely to be released some day. Treatment for the offender at the time was mostly psychoanalytically based despite the fact that such therapy was designed for people with very different problems. I had my doubts about the efficacy of such general therapy for sex offenders, and later research would confirm my fears. Insight therapy produces sex offenders with insight, but they're still sex offenders, and they continue offending. At the time, however, I knew nothing better to do than traditional therapy.

Eventually, I got annoyed. Annoyed at what a lousy job I and everybody else seemed to be doing with sexual abuse. I got tired of violence, tired of entitled and predatory people getting away with everything short of murder—and sometimes that as well. And being born a Southerner, I got stubborn.

I began to look around the country for more effective therapies, for better ways that treatment providers could work with the criminal justice system. And I began to study sex offenders, to talk to them and to listen. It struck me that many of the books I was reading sounded as though the authors had never spoken to a sex offender. So I began to interview offenders, and eventually I wrote books and made educational films of them talking about their crimes and their ways of getting access to victims.

It's now more than twenty years later, and I know a little more than I knew in the beginning. Also, there is now an entire field of study about sex offenders whereas before there wasn't much of anything. This book is largely not about that research, although I make reference to it. It is also not a book about pedophilic priests, although I talk about that problem as well. This book is a more personal account of what I've learned from sitting in rooms with predators.

It is, first of all, a book about secrecy and deception because secrecy is the lifeblood of sexual aggression. It is a book about why and how sex offenders get away with their crimes for decades, sometimes forever. It is about how they fool you and me and people like us everywhere. It will touch on why we are so trusting, which we are as long as the offender isn't poor and toothless and/or of a different ethnic group, as long as he looks like us and talks like us—most certainly if he's a priest or pediatrician or teacher.

This is not a book with complete and comfortable answers. It will not finish with a checklist for identifying a sex offender: Just add up the points, and you too can spot your neighborhood pedophile or rapist. But if I do my job right, reading this book will make it harder for sex offenders to get access to you or your children. It will make it harder because knowing how they think and act and operate is the best protection that we have. Indeed, it is the only protection that is possible.

Buy all the guns you want, but guns will not likely help you. Sex offenders only very rarely sneak into a house in the middle of the night. More often they come through the front door in the day, as friends and neighbors, as Boy Scout leaders, priests, principals, teachers, doctors, and coaches. They are invited into our homes time after time, and we give them permission to take our children on the overnight camping trip, the basketball game, or down to the Salvation Army post for youth activities.

We give permission because we don't recognize these people as predators, because we think sex offenders are monsters and surely we would recognize a monster, wouldn't we? That nice young minister who runs all the youth programs, the one with the crooked smile and the thatch of brown hair over his brow, the one who visits the elderly and gives the poor money from his own funds—surely not him. He could not be a child molester with ninety victims while he's still in his twenties. That good-looking, polite young man who just wants to see the motorcycle for sale in the back yard. Surely he couldn't be a rapist with a knife in his hip pocket waiting for you to turn your back to pull the cover off.

I sit in rooms with such men, and they tell me their side of the story. They tell me what you don't see, about the thoughts and feelings and hungers that drive them. They tell me how they operate and how they got away with assaults for so long. They tell me how they make assessments of people like you and me. I get to see, sometimes, the face we don't see in public.

Why me? Not because I have any magic to get them to talk, only that I am often talking to them after the conviction and sentencing, and they know nothing they say will hurt them legally. As a condition of their talking, I agree to report what they say anonymously. In any case, they know better than to give me the kinds of details needed to prosecute. The truth is that many sex offenders like to talk about their exploits—if it can be done in some way that doesn't hurt them in court. They are proud of what clever fellows they are. Narcissism is their Achilles' heel.

And narcissism has caused a number of them to agree to be involved in educational films I have made on sex offenders.[2] Because I taped a number of sex offenders for those films, I have transcripts of the tapes, which formed the basis of many of the quotes you will see throughout this book.[3]

I have not found it all that easy to sit in rooms listening to sex offenders talk about child molestation, rape, and even torture—particularly torture. It was certainly never a dream of mine growing up, to be a specialist in violence and mayhem. I spent most of my adolescence on a basketball court, practicing fade away jumpers and setting picks. The only violence I was interested in occurred under the boards. If you had tapped that skinny fourteen-year-old on the shoulder and told her she would grow up to work with sex offenders, she would have told you that you had the wrong girl. There weren't many white girls in the 1950s growing up in the South who wanted to be Bill Russell when they grew up, but I surely did. Still do, for that matter.

But the violence I see now is a long way from a basketball court, and I have discovered there is a price to be paid for seeing it. Once in a three-day taping that included several sadists, the material was so overwhelming that both the film crew and I got sick—I with a sinus infection, and the entire film crew with a flu so severe they had to delay their departure from the motel. Our immune systems had weakened, I believe, from the beating our souls had taken.

Malevolence takes a bite out of your spirit. Just sitting with it, just talking with people who consciously and deliberately exploit others, feels like being beaten. Over the years, I have seen many therapists burn out and leave the field entirely. Even though I have stayed, I have become less trusting than most, more protective of my children (some would say more paranoid) in general.

But if what I know hurts me personally and affects my life in ways I am not happy about, it still feels like work that needs to be done. It is precisely our lack of knowledge and understanding that gives predators their edge, and there's nothing wrong with trying to level the playing field a little. What follows is an attempt to describe, to make meaning of what I've seen in the course of two decades, to make sense of harm's way.

1

The Problem

"A. A violent order is disorder; and
B. A great disorder is an order, These
Two things are one."[1]

The woman across from me has a lyrical voice that is mesmerizing. This voice should have been singing lullabies to a sleepless preschooler, not talking about locking her children in the bedroom while her husband and his father broke down the door to her apartment with machetes.

She is sitting across from me because I am known as an expert on sex offenders, sadists in particular. Emma[2] is not my client; I am not her therapist. The prosecutor who made sure her husband was civilly committed as a sexually violent predator has arranged for me to talk to her. We are both there for the same reason. She wants to learn more about sadists so that she can make sense of her ex-husband and her life. She wants to talk to an "expert." I want to learn more about sadists so that I can become better at evaluating them and testifying against them. I want to talk to an expert too. But only one of us is talking to a real expert.

Surely, I could *claim* to be the expert in the room. I have a Ph.D. in psychology from Harvard and have given lectures on sex offenders in more than forty states and in ten countries. I have given keynote addresses at national conferences on the topic in four of those countries. In 1997 I won the Significant Achievement Award of the Association of the Treatment of Sexual Abusers, given to one person in the world every year. I have made educational films on the topic and have written two academic books, one of which has gone into fifteen printings and has been called the Bible of sex offender treatment. I even write mysteries about sex offenders based on my experience in the field. But my credentials pale next to Emma's.

You'd be surprised at the times he's at my bed. I see him standing in the doorway, the way he was when I tried to get away from him. He'd always find me. He'd climb through my windows. He beat me with a clothes hanger, and he cut me with a knife when I moved.

This man has taken thirty-one years of my life away from me. I'm forty-seven. Thirty-one years he's taken from me. He's always going to be tomorrow. He's always going to be tomorrow. The only way I'll ever get rid of him and what he's done to me is die. And even in death I feel somewhere in those last few minutes, those last few seconds he's going to be right there.

I do not argue. I do not tell her tomorrow will be a better day or that time can heal anything. I do not tell her he will not be there in the last few seconds before she dies. I am a Southerner, and my grandmother taught me to know the sound of "gospel truth" when I hear it.

I can answer some of her questions, and I can tell her I believe her. Odd how important that is to her, given how much corroborating material there is in the records. But she still does not expect to be believed, despite her ex-husband's murder conviction in a different state, despite the fact that he killed his victim in front of the victim's four-year-old daughter, raped the child, turned on the gas, and left the child to die (which she refused to do).

Emma leans forward and tilts her head inquisitively, "What makes people be like that?" she says. That question is why she's here. It is the one she wants answered.

It is an important question, and it deserves a decent answer. Theories and research flit through my head, odd studies that show that psychopaths don't respond the same way to emotional words as other people. For most of us, emotional words are recognized faster than neutral words. For psychopaths, they are recognized more slowly. It is as if they are more fundamental and more meaningful for most people; for psychopaths it's as if they are a second language.

The rest of us blink more when we're startled in the middle of viewing something unpleasant. Why is that? Who knows? But maybe the aversiveness of something unpleasant puts our nervous system on red alert. Being tense already, it reacts more when startled. Nothing like that happens to psychopaths. Landscapes. Burn victims. There's not much difference from their point of view.

There is a lot of research on psychopaths, and much of it is very worrisome: studies, for example, that show that the quality of parenting is unrelated to the number of conduct problems that callous/unemotional children have. From the start they seem to be on a set trajectory that even good parenting won't change. The research flitting through my head goes on and on as I try to come up with an answer. I think of the biological theories and the sociological theories and the learning theories. Finally, I say simply, "The truth is, we don't really know."

Emma looks disappointed. After all, she thinks she's talking to an expert. And now it is my turn to ask the question that matters to me, the one I know will be hard to answer.

"How did you finally get away?"

She tries to answer. "I acted like a crazy person. I went to his mom's house and I shot it up," she says. Then she pauses. "When you ask me a question like that, there's no simple answer. There's no simple answers to anything that has to do with Avery."

She tries again. "It started with those girls, those last two girls." She is referring to two girls Avery kidnapped and held captive at the house, the two girls he beat and raped along with her, always raping one and making the others watch. The last two girls.

It is a hard question for her to answer, how she finally got out of it. But through the stories she tells, I hear this: She got to the point where she no longer cared if she lived or died, where threats had no power and where she no longer felt the beatings. She had to get so crazy she was uncontrollable. It got to the point where he had to kill her or let her go. It could have gone either way.

Still she got away. Sort of. He is always there, she says again, standing by her bed.

It was never Emma's choice to marry this man or even to get involved with him. At age fifteen she was pregnant by a young man in her church. When she told her mother, a mother who had never been kind to her, she responded that Emma was lying; no young man in the church would do anything like that. Soon after that, Emma was playing tag football in the street, and she ran out for a pass. A man who hung around with her brother at car races ran up to her. "Your mama said I could have you," he told her, "so I'm gonna marry you." Emma just kept running for the pass.

She should have just kept on going. Just headed down the street and never looked back. But Emma had no clue what was in store with the man who had claimed her and besides, there was no place to go. So she did what her mama told her. She married him. Even before the marriage took place, he started beating her. After the marriage, he beat her every day, pregnant or not. In her mind, he still does.

Emma's story ought to be rarer than it is. You and I should be able to pick up a local newspaper without seeing a new charge of child molestation against somebody in our area. Catholics should not be afraid to let their children be altar boys. Parents should not be worried about overnight camp. I should meet many people who do not know anyone personally who has been raped or molested as a child. But I can't remember seeing a newspaper without a rape or molestation charge in it somewhere, and when I ask groups how many people know someone personally with a history of molestation, almost always, every hand in the room goes up.

Research has not been slow to document how frequently sexual assaults occur in this country. We have just been slow to pay attention. Researchers beginning in 1929 documented rates of sexual abuse of female children that ranged from 24 percent to 37 percent.[3] Research on males has been rarer, but what research there has been found alarming rates, somewhere between 27 percent and 30 percent.[4]

These older studies lacked the sophisticated methodology of more modern research, and their definitions of sexual abuse were less precise. No doubt some of what they defined as sexual abuse would be considered normal sex play between children today. Still, the examples given in these studies make it clear that much of it, indeed, was sexual abuse.

What is most striking is that these studies documented what was surely thought to be sexual abuse at the time, yet no one paid attention.

Modern research has confirmed what early researchers found. Dr. Gene Abel and colleagues conducted studies of sex offenders in the late 1980s that asked voluntary sex offender clients how many total offenses they had committed.[5] The studies guaranteed confidentiality in a variety of ways: The interviewers did not have the subjects' names, only their research numbers; they had obtained a federal certificate of confidentiality that blocked the results from being subpoenaed into any federal court in this country; the master list was kept outside the country in any case.[6]

Results stunned the professional community. Two hundred and thirty-two child molesters admitted attempting more than fifty-five thousand incidents of molestation. They claimed to have been successful in 38,000 incidents and reported they had more than 17,000 total victims. All this from only 232 men. Men who molested out-of-home female children averaged twenty victims. Although there were fewer of them, men who molested out-of-home male children were even more active than molesters of female children, averaging 150 victims each.

Dr. Abel also analyzed the data for all kinds of sex offenses, including exhibitionism, voyeurism, and adult rape as well as child molestation. This larger sample of 561 offenders admitted to more than 291,000 sexual offenses of all kinds and more than 195,000 victims.

It is difficult to appreciate just how large a number 195,000 is, but consider that the Louisiana Superdome, site of five Super Bowls, has a maximum seating capacity of 72,675. If all the victims of those 561 men wanted to meet, they would have filled two and one-half Superdomes.

Despite the astounding figures, most of these offenses had never been detected. In fact, Abel computed the chances of being caught for a sexual offense at 3 percent. Crime pays, it seems, and sexual crime pays particularly well.

But how do we know these men aren't lying? Bragging about things that never happened? Unfortunately, studies of victims confirm what offenders say. In a classic study of adult women in the general population, Dr. Diana Russell found—and later research by Dr. Gail Wyatt and others confirmed—that rates of child sexual abuse are extraordinarily high.[7] Twenty-eight percent of Russell's sample of women had been molested as children under the age of fourteen, 38 percent if the fourteen- through seventeen-year-olds are included. These were physical contact offenses only—exhibitionism was not counted—and they excluded nonviolent sexual contact between peers. Nonetheless, only 5 percent of the child sexual abuse revealed to these researchers had ever been reported to the authorities.

Figures on males show lower but still alarming rates. Although male-oriented pedophiles are highly active, there are fewer of them than there are of men who molest female children. Nonetheless, between 9 and 16 percent of boys in the United States are likely to be molested before they reach adulthood.[8]

These are figures for child molestation, but Russell found the figures on adult rape to be no comfort either.[9] Forty-one percent of women in the Russell study had either been the victims of rape or of attempted rape as adults. If spousal rape was included, the number went up to 44 percent. Research by Dr. Mary Koss and others documents that between 15 and 27 percent of female college students are the victims of rape or attempted rape by the time they leave college.[10]

Methodologically sound studies of *completed* rather than attempted rape produce figures in the general population that range from 12.7 percent to 24 percent,[11] with two studies finding intermediate rates of 15 percent and 20 percent, respectively.[12] The higher figures are truly frightening, and unfortunately Russell's work—which found the higher rates—is still the most rigorous of the group.

But even the lower rates are distressing. Even if the very lowest study is correct—which is not likely—it means that, minimally, one in every nine women in this country will be raped at some point in her life, which in itself is a dreadful figure.

The dry research figures only confirm what I have seen over and over in this field: There are a lot of sexual offenses out there, and the people who commit them don't get caught very often. When an offender is caught and has a thorough evaluation with a polygraph backup, he will reveal dozens, sometimes hundreds, of offenses for which he was never apprehended. In an unpublished study by psychologist Dr. Pamela Van Wyk, twenty-three offenders in her incarcerated treatment program entered the program admitting an average of three victims each. Faced with a polygraph and the necessity of passing it to stay in the treatment program, they revealed an average of 175 victims each.

A recent article by therapist Jan Hindman summarized a series of three studies she conducted in different time periods, each comparing polygraph to no polygraph in terms of how many victims offenders revealed.[13] Although the absolute numbers were less than those above, the number of victims revealed with the threat of a polygraph (and conditional immunity from prosecution for the disclosures) was four to six times as many as were revealed without the polygraph.

And these are only the offenders who were caught. In treating victims since 1978, I have heard the stories over and over of offenders who were *never* caught. A young woman tells me that as a young teen, she and a friend were raped repeatedly by a friend of their parents. It went on for years. He would rape the girls in front of each other and threatened the lives of both of them if they told. They didn't. They were both afraid of him and convinced they wouldn't be believed anyway, given his high standing in the community and his friendship with their parents. There is a song she still hates, she tells me, because he used to sing it as he undressed them.

Her friend committed suicide as a young adult. My client has been plagued with low self-esteem, ongoing nightmares, and depression. She has always lived a walled-off existence, keeping others at emotional arms' length.

And what happened to him, I ask? "Him?" she says, perplexed at the question. "Nothing. He's still moderator of the town meetings." There, in a town less than fifty miles from the small New England town I was living in at the time, was a predator who was bold enough to rape children in front of each other. He was implicated in the suicide of one, had damaged the life of another, and more than a decade later was standing up in front of his peers cracking jokes. And, no doubt, still singing his song.

In all the interviews I have done, I cannot remember one offender who did not admit privately to more victims than those for whom he had been caught. On the contrary, most offenders had been charged with and/or convicted of from one to three victims. In the interviews I have done, they have admitted to roughly 10 to 1,250 victims. What was truly frightening was that all the offenders had been reported before by children, and the reports had been ignored.

Ignoring a valid disclosure can have disastrous results. At the least, it increases an offender's confidence in his ability to get away with it. Often, it is a license to reoffend against that same child. One molester told me

I believed if they told, that their mother or father wouldn't believe them. And when I found out that they didn't, I would go back and molest or rape them again.

But not all children tell in the first place. For reasons as varied as fear of the offender, shame at their helplessness, love and protection of a parent, or even—if the offender is clever enough to stroke their genitals—shame of their own sexual arousal during the sex acts—they don't tell.

Also, they often think their silence affects only them. One man reported that as a child, he had thought there was something wrong with him that made his principal choose him. He must be gay, he thought, or somehow he had done something that caused the principal to "punish" him with abuse. The reality never broke over him until twenty years later when he returned to the town as an adult and saw the principal ride by with another twelve-year-old in the car. In all those years he had never once considered that the principal might be a risk to other children. This man is hard on himself for not revealing the abuse. He feels now it would have protected other children, and, of course, he assumes it would have protected him from further abuse. I wish I believed either of those were true.

2

Deception

I stare at the child's statement in front of me. It is a report by a social worker of a four-year-old's account of sexual abuse by her father:

> During my interview with Julie, she was able to identify all the body parts of a stuffed teddy bear. She referred to the bear's rear end as his "bottom" and referred to its genital area as his "peepee." At one point during the interview Julie stated that her dad licked and sucked her peepee and that she sucked his peepee. She further stated that when her dad sucked her peepee he made her peepee sting.
>
> Julie said her dad did this in the bedroom with the blinds shut and under the covers. She said this happened when she was four-years-old and her mother was not there. Julie stated that she would tell her dad to stop sucking her peepee.
>
> Julie stated that her father would take her nightgown off and lick her peepee. She said it felt good for a little while and then it would sting.

I consider the report carefully. It is filled with detail. The words are a child's words, the description exact. It is clear this child knows what oral sex is. It shows no signs of coaching. But why was this report sent to me with all identifying information removed by a polygrapher I barely know? I read on through the foot or so of accompanying information in the file.

This report, I learn, surfaced in the middle of a custody fight. Dad was a wealthy businessman, successful, well respected, and well liked. Mom was an inpatient in a drug unit. My heart sinks. It does not matter how realistic this report is, how many signs of credibility, how few signs of coaching. In our system of justice, lawyers are for sale. Dad's money is going to buy some very good lawyers indeed. It isn't clear that Mom has either the money or the will to oppose him. And the child—she'll be lucky to be represented at all. I've thought many times that if I were accused of a crime, I'd rather have the better lawyer than be innocent.

But it is not so simple, it seems. The court responds appropriately and appoints two independent psychologists to make a recommendation. Two independent chances to get it right. Two people who are not beholden to either side and who can ask for any test, even a polygraph, as part of their decision-making. Two people whose job it is to know something about deception and to sort out the true from the false.

But both psychologists opt instead for what is termed an "interactional assessment." They simply watch the father interact with his daughter, looking for signs of bonding or, conversely, fear. They believe if he abused her, she will be afraid of him; if she loves him, he is innocent.

Of course, there is no research and no good theory to support this approach. I stood up in a conference once when someone was discussing this type of assessment and noted the lack of research to support it. I mentioned that sex offenders are notorious for bonding with a child and using that relationship to manipulate the child into having sex with them. I stated that, in addition, a child might be afraid of the man for entirely different reasons. Perhaps he beat her mother but never laid a hand on her. What justification did the presenters have for believing that one could tell from the interaction between child and alleged perpetrator whether the abuse had occurred or not? The speaker turned to a colleague in the audience and said, "Help me out, will you?"

In this child's case, the alleged perpetrator is the child's father. Surely she loves him, even if he did what she has disclosed. He has not used violence. She does not necessarily know there is anything wrong with what he's doing. She is four years old. One of the evaluators notes, "Observations of father and daughter indicate a very happy, spontaneous and positive relationship." I sigh. As if that had anything to do with anything. The fact that she loves him doesn't mean that he's innocent or guilty. Then I find something that makes me sit up straight.

> Of concern are the admissions by Mr. Jones that earlier in his life he had engaged in sexually inappropriate behavior with three children. . . . These were the children of the woman he was living with at the time.

I stare at the note. This psychologist knew he'd done it before—in identical circumstances. It is a damning admission and surely means the psychologist should take this latest disclosure seriously. But he does not. Mr. Jones, it seems, is too charming, too rich, too respected. Despite knowing he is an admitted child molester, both psychologists recommend that full custody go to Dad.

And there the story ends—in most such cases. But the attorney for the father, convinced his man was innocent, sent him to a polygrapher. I know he thought he was innocent because he sent him to a very good polygrapher—not the man to whom one would knowingly send a guilty client. This polygrapher is an unusually good interrogator and has a 98 percent confession rate for people who test deception on his polygraph. I have seen him present at the yearly conference of the American Polygraph Association, and I know his techniques. I have heard him describe what he says to his clients:

> Now the problem with the polygraph is that it can't tell the difference in a big lie and a little lie and I would hate, I would truly hate for you to mess up your polygraph with something little that don't amount to a hill of beans. So if there is *anything, anything* at all that you want to tell me before the polygraph, now's the time so we can get it out of the way.

Under these instructions, the polygrapher found that Mr. Jones had quite a few things to say:

> She grabs his penis while he washes her in the shower, and he has

explained to her what a man does with it. When questioned further about how often this happens, he said three or four times a week. When asked to give a high figure regarding the number of times that Julie has touched his penis, he said about twenty times.

The polygraph report goes on:

He also acknowledges erections and masturbating in the shower while Julie is in the shower with him and acknowledged that on about five occasions that he can recall, she has played with his penis while it is erect, stating this is educational for her.

"Letting" Julie fondle him is a direct admission of child sexual abuse. But that's not all. The report goes on:

Her father stated that he sleeps nude and stated that Julie likes to cuddle. He stated she likes to run her foot up and down his penis until he gets an erection and sometimes "things happen."

Once he starts, Mr. Jones seems more than happy to talk. He tells the polygrapher about his use of vibrators on the child:

He stated that she "loves" to orgasm. "I'll get her a vibrator. She'll hold the handle against her peepee and giggle until she climaxes."

All these statements occurred before Mr. Jones even took the polygraph. He has openly admitted to child sexual abuse. In addition to all that he admits beforehand, he fails the polygraph. What he does not admit—not until after he fails the polygraph—is oral sex. In the dry language of the report, Mr. Jones finally comes clean:

She has licked and sucked on his penis no more than five times, has given him two full "blow jobs." He has "69ed" her. He has licked her vagina and has performed oral sex on her not more than ten times.

In a note, the polygrapher mentions that Mr. Jones complained that Julie was so small that it hurt his back when he "69ed" her. Perhaps I can be forgiven for thinking prison would do wonders for Mr. Jones's back.

But it is not to be. And I know that, even as I turn the pages searching for the disposition of the case. I have been in this field too long to think that just because the man is guilty and just because someone got the truth out of him automatically means he was held accountable.

I find a handwritten note from the polygrapher in the file. He faxed the report to the attorney for the father. It was a private polygraph, after all, requested by the father's attorney and not one required by either of the independent evaluators. Within five minutes of faxing the report, the phone rang, "I've worked with you for twenty years," the attorney said to him. "I hope I don't have to remind you what privileged communication means."

What privileged communication means is that this report fell under attorney-client privilege and therefore was suppressed. What it means is that the father's attorney was under *no* requirement whatsoever to release the report to the court, and, by law, the polygrapher could not. To do so would have been a violation of the father's rights—the polygraph was done for the father's attorney, after all. The report, had the polygrapher sent it to the court, would have cost the polygrapher his license to practice and still never would have been admitted into evidence.

What it means is that the only reports the court saw in this case were by the two psychologists who thought they could tell whether the father was lying by interviewing him and that they could tell if the child was abused by seeing if she loved her father. What it means was that in 1996, full custody of this child went to her father, where it has remained ever since.

I close the papers. The polygrapher, anguished by the outcome, sent them to me after removing the real names, with the hope that I can use them for "educational purposes." So I do. But first I have to deal with that knot in my stomach. I have long understood that we cannot save every child from the subterranean river of misery that flows through so many childhoods. I acknowledge it. Most days I accept it as the way things are. Most days.

The problem is deception. Despite the fact that decades of research have demonstrated that people cannot reliably tell who's lying and who isn't,[1] most people believe they can. There is something so fundamentally threatening about the notion that we cannot really know whether or not to trust someone that it is very difficult to get anyone—clinicians, citizens, even police—to take such results seriously.

Whereas the polygrapher in the Jones case has nightmares about the child he could not help, the two independent evaluators—either one of whom could have asked for a polygraph that could *not* have been suppressed—likely feel all too sure of their findings. How could they not? Mr. Jones was a well-respected member of the community with a crazy wife. And he was so sincere. Clearly, the child loved him dearly. Besides, look at all the character references he had. Such a man is hardly likely to be a child molester, now is he?

This is not an isolated case. I remember a case in which the child's account was so specific and so credible that the evaluator could not fault it. She wrote:

> Jonathan [4 years old] has exhibited behaviors which are consistent with behaviors experienced by children who have been sexually abused. . . . Also, according to both parents, he spontaneously reported the abuse incident without any apparent coaching from other adults. Each parent stated that Margaret [Jonathan's mother and former wife of the alleged perpetrator] did not have a reason to coach Jonathan. . . . Jonathan was very clear in his description of what happened and showed consistent affect, including anger and sadness. . . . Jonathan's statements were consistent regarding "who" he named as the perpetrator and the specific event.

Nonetheless, the examiner concluded that she could not determine the identity of the perpetrator—even though she believed Jonathan had been sexually abused and despite the fact that his father was the only offender that Jonathan ever named.

What evidence did she offer that Jonathan may have been abused by a different perpetrator and not the one he consistently named?

Since his father denied these allegations, it is difficult to determine the identity of the perpetrator. In support of Mr. Hagen's truthfulness . . . he was very forthright during the interview and testing procedures. For example, he acknowledged having difficulty in his sexual relations at times, and he openly admitted that he had a possible drinking problem in his past.

Because he admitted some problems, she concluded he would not lie about other more serious problems. Because he admitted problems that were legal, she concluded he would not lie about activity that was illegal. Of course, that is just a made-up reason. The truth is, she simply believed him.

It happens all the time—to professionals at least as much as to the general public. A man was arrested for a series of rapes and sent to a therapist for a psycho-sexual evaluation. The therapist's report describes the two of them walking to the office. The man "stayed back to close one of the doors, a very solicitous gesture that, as it turned out, is consistent with his general pattern of behavior." The report went on to describe him as "kind, thoughtful, and considerate, a person who seemed to take pleasure in helping and caring." Instead of concluding that: 1) the man knew better than to backhand his wife in the office during a court-ordered interview; and 2) he was good at putting up a front, the evaluator concluded that the man must not be a serial rapist—damn the eyewitness accounts. Serial rapists, after all, are brutal, and this man was not brutal in the office. Therefore, he wasn't brutal outside of it. Fortunately, there was considerable evidence that he was guilty, and he was convicted. The court got it right even if the psychologist did not.

Even treatment centers that specialize in treating sex offenders can be astonishingly naïve. One of the priest cases I have testified in was in

1994 in which the offender, whom I will call Father Drover, was sent to a center set up by the Catholic church for the treatment of pedophilic priests. This particular offender arrived with a known history of sexual offenses against adolescent boys. In his records were: 1) an accusation of sexual abuse by a fourteen-year-old boy in 1983; 2) a conviction for trying to solicit sex from a fourteen-year-old boy in 1988; and 3) another accusation of sexual abuse by a young teenager whom Father Drover saw in his role as counselor. Father Drover also came with two evaluations, both of which saw him as a serious risk to reoffend, and one of which called him a "fixated sexual offender, a man who has a primary sexual interest in children."

Father Drover, however, was a personable and charming man, and before long the treatment center had accepted his version of events. In Father's Drover version, one of the molestations consisted simply of his kissing a boy who was sitting in his lap, whereas the second was a fabrication by a boy who asked him for sex, but Father Drover refused. The boy then retaliated by falsely accusing him of abuse. As for the conviction for solicitation, what had really happened was that the boy offered to "do anything for money," whereas Father Drover had simply warned him that he would get in trouble for saying something like that. Father Drover pled guilty, the treatment center concluded, only to spare the church.

After a brief course of "treatment," the center declared the previous evaluations dead wrong about Father Drover's interest in young adolescent boys. They noted that "he had a depth of conscientiousness and sensitivity to others, and a very high degree of ethical concern that did not fit with what the reports said of him." In fact, they felt so strongly that he was not a pedophile that they hired him to be on their staff.

Later, after Father Drover was charged with eighteen additional counts of sexual abuse and was accused by four more victims, the people at the treatment center still refused to believe he was a child molester. Father Drover had "clearly stated his innocence to us, and we believed him—and continue to believe him," they said in court documents. They maintained he was "totally honest in his therapeutic process" and believed "his progress was excellent and his recovery work was commendable." He would "not be a risk to society or himself in terms of sexually acting out." The staff at the treatment center said all this even though the reports clearly showed that the abuse he was being charged with had occurred before he went into their program, which meant that everything he had told them was a lie.

In fact, interviews with the boys and their court testimony made it clear Father Drover was an extremely fixated pedophile and an unusually callous one. He had repeatedly befriended children—often from poor or troubled families—who were in counseling with him, and he lavished gifts, presents, and affection on them. Then he would molest them in callous and sometimes brutal ways.

For example, one boy was crying in a counseling session about his increasing drug problem and his family difficulties. Father Grover got up, undid the boy's pants, and started performing fellatio on him. On another occasion, he was performing fellatio on a boy when he suddenly left the room. Another priest came in and finished the job. On yet another occasion, he took a boy to a rectory for an overnight visit where two other men were allowed to anally rape the boy that night. There were other children he was molesting during their confirmation counseling sessions, when he would also try to persuade them to prostitute themselves with strangers for money. He molested three brothers in the same family. Many of the children he molested were in counseling for emotional or drug and alcohol problems.

Sometimes the naivety of professionals can be fatal. A very well-known psychologist in a state where I once worked evaluated a three-month-old infant with bite marks all over him. Only two people had the opportunity to inflict the bites within the time frame, and they were the parents. Suspicion centered on the father, and the psychologist was asked to evaluate him. She reported how tenderly he wiped the infant's nose in the evaluation, how carefully he held the baby. Based on the man's behavior in the interview, she exonerated him and recommended custody remain with the parents. Two years later he killed the child.

This is an issue that will never die. It seems impossible to convince people that private behavior cannot be predicted from public behavior. Kind, nonviolent individuals behave well in public, but so do many people who are brutal behind the scenes. Even as I write these words, I am embroiled in a case in which an adolescent was accused of sexually abusing a child in his mother's home day care several years ago. Social services founded the case, which is to say they considered the case genuine, but unaccountably did not revoke the mother's day care license. Other parents, not knowing that there was an adolescent with a substantiated case of child sexual abuse against him in the home, continued to send their children to the day care.

Just recently he abused another child. He anally raped a three-year-old so violently that he tore a hole in her anus. The quarter-size tear dumped sufficient bacteria into her abdominal cavity that she died within twenty-four hours of the assault.

There were two police jurisdictions involved, the one in which the teen lived and the one in which the victim lived. The police who knew him and his family decided this teen was far too nice to have done this, although the police who didn't know him and only had the evidence disagreed. The medical examiner unaccountably asked for an interview with the teen and softened his report afterward to say that perhaps the tear expanded as the infection progressed. Perhaps it was just a nick at first, say, from a fingernail. Just the simple insertion of a fingernail, nothing really violent, the report implied. He also stated in his testimony that this teen did not fit the profile of a child molester, although one wonders how much experience a pathologist has with child molester profiles (which don't exist in any case). An independent psychologist who was appointed by the court to evaluate the teen told the judge bluntly that "you've got the wrong defendant."

What makes this most perplexing is that while all these professionals agreed the teen was innocent, the teen in fact confessed. He confessed not through a lengthy, exhausting interview or by being threatened, but when he was simply told they were running DNA tests on him (a bluff—they did not have material to analyze).

The judge in his decision gave something to both sides. He found the teen guilty of sexual assault but not of homicide. Because it was absolutely established that the sexual assault led to the child's death, it was an astonishing decision. If the teen was guilty of the sexual assault, then he killed her. If he did not kill her, it can only be because he was not guilty of the sexual assault. I shake my head in wonder. The judge could not ignore the valid confession the teen gave. On the other hand, he must have believed something that the professionals told him. All I know is this: If social services had pulled the day care license when the first report was substantiated, the three-year-old would be alive today.

Recently I interviewed a psychopath. This is always a humbling experience because it teaches me over and over how much of human motivation and experience is outside my narrow range. Despite the psychopath's lack of conscience and lack of empathy for others, he is inevitably better at fooling people than any other type of offender. I suppose a conscience just slows people down. A convicted child molester, this particular one made friends with a correctional officer who invited him to live in his home after he was released—invited him despite the fact the officer had a nine-year-old daughter.

The officer and his wife were so taken with the offender that, after the offender lived with them for a few months, they initiated adoption proceedings—adoption for a man almost their age. Of course, he was a child molester living in the same house as a child. Not surprisingly, he molested the daughter the entire time he lived there. Later, when this was disclosed and the offender was reincarcerated, the guard and his wife continued to try to visit him in prison. They wanted to understand how he could do this. They wanted to see him. They were still attached to him. Even the offender was astonished by their behavior. He told his psychologist, "I feel like saying, 'What the fuck is wrong with you, lady. I molested your fucking daughter.'"

The saddest part of this story is that if this offender weren't tired of toying with the guard and his wife, he could easily do it again. All he would have to do is cry and feign regret, and in all likelihood the guard and his wife would shortly be advocating for the inmate's release with the parole board.

What these experiences have taught me is that even when people are warned by a previously founded case or even a conviction, they still routinely underestimate the pathology with which they are dealing.

Niceness and likability will override a track record of child molestation any day of the week.

Likability is such a potent weapon that it protects predators for long periods of time and through almost incomprehensible numbers of victims. Mr. Saylor, an athletic director in an elementary school, operated undisturbed for almost twenty years. He tells me there is almost no limit to the number of molestations that one can get away with.

I created my first victim when I was thirteen, a female victim. . . . Sally was six and I was thirteen, and I raped and molested Sally by forcing my hands and fingers on her vulva and in her vagina and forcing objects into her vagina. Sally is my only female victim, my one female victim. I created my first male victim when I was fifteen, and I have been victimizing male children virtually nonstop until my incarceration.

Q. How old are you now?

A. I'm thirty-three now, and I have been incarcerated for three years. . . .

Q. How many total victims did you have?

A. I have eleven male rape victims, one female rape victim, and I have approximately 1,250 male molest victims, and I say approximately because I really don't know.

I am stunned by this number and fumble around for a few minutes. Finally I find my voice.

Q. How many kids were you molesting a week to have a rate like that?

A. There were times when I went a whole week, two weeks, three weeks without ever molesting anybody. And there were other times that I molested daily. Two and three times a day. On average I would say I molested five children a week over that twenty year period. . . .

Q. And you mean five different kids?

A. Yes.

There were several outcries by children over the years, but it was not easy for parents to accept that a man with Mr. Saylor's impeccable credentials and otherwise responsible behavior might be molesting children.

One child's family, by no means atypical, simply said to their son, "John loves you. John wouldn't do anything to hurt you. There must be some mistake." Mr. Saylor told me the child made no mistake at all. It took almost twenty years and well over a thousand child victims before a single allegation stuck.

Such a long period of molesting without consequences changed Mr. Saylor.

After so many years of raping and molesting, I finally reached a point to where it was like I felt invincible. The children love me. They care about me. They're not going to tell regardless of what I do. And my thinking was also, even if they do tell, based on past conditions which parents did not believe the children, my thinking was they're not going to believe the child anyway, and I got very bold with my molest. . . .

There is no . . . Let me rephrase that. There were no boundaries for me. No place was off limits. No time was off limits. And no set of circumstances was off limits. At any time that I saw an opportunity to get what I wanted, which was to rape or molest, I took advantage of it.

There were other times that I molested and raped while at work. Or I simply manipulated the child into coming into my office, and I just simply locked the door and proceeded to do what I wanted to do, which was to rape the child.

My nephew, I raped him for a period of nine years. Raped and molested him for a period of nine years. And very few cases did I rape him in which no one was in the house.

I sit silent for a moment, thinking. How many mothers over the years have I heard testify that he *couldn't* have molested their child? They were always present.

Did they ever sleep? I would ask. They would always look at me incredulously. How could anyone get up in the night and molest a child without the other parent knowing? After all, they always assure me, they are very light sleepers. But I have had victims and offenders both tell me of offenders who molested children while the wife was sleeping in the same bed. That Mr. Saylor would molest a child in an office adjacent to a gym full of people does not surprise me. I have seen an interview with an offender who talked about leaving the door open and molesting a child with his wife in the next room. The possibility of getting caught just added to the thrill.

But still, Mr. Saylor does manage to surprise me, for he has done something I have never seen before.

There were times that I raped in a car with the parents in the front seat, me in the backseat with the children. The child would feel such a bond of trust that the child would decide okay, I'd like to go to sleep, and I'd manipulate the child and lay him across the seat and molest the child with my hand on his penis. By forcing my hands on his penis while the parents were in the front seat.

Why would a child not tell? Because, for reasons we do not clearly understand, children freeze when confronted with something they cannot make sense of. A child in the back seat with an adult's hand on his penis is not going to know how to understand or explain that. He will think that an adult whom he loves and respects can't be doing anything wrong. Besides, this is an adult *his parents* respect. He will likely wonder if his parents even know and approve. After all, they're in the front seat. Or he'll be embarrassed and wonder if he will be blamed.

Regardless of the reason, the fact seems undeniable. It is only a minority of children who disclose abuse at the time.[2] No study I can find on this topic has ever found otherwise.

If children can be silenced and the average person is easy to fool, many offenders report that religious people are even easier to fool than most people. One molester, who was himself a minister, said:

I considered church people easy to fool . . . they have a trust that comes from being Christians. . . . They tend to be better folks all around. And they seem to want to believe in the good that exists in all people. . . . I think they want to believe in people. And because of that, you can easily convince, with or without convincing words.

In interviewing victims in the growing number of cases involving priests, I have been surprised—although I should not have been—by how deeply religious many of the victims' families were. I had never before grasped that it was the most religious families who were thrilled to have a priest take an interest in their children, who wanted their children to be altar boys, who could not believe that a priest would do anything so wrong.

The growing crisis in the Catholic Church just underlines the fact that offenders can recognize ideal settings for child molesters even if the rest of us can't. In truth, a deeply religious and trusting group of people, plus the requirement of celibacy (an ideal cover for any man who has no sexual interest in adults), plus a hierarchy that doesn't report complaints to the police and simply moves the offender on to new and fresh territory with new potential victims, is the ideal setting for pedophiles. Even without such extreme conditions, however, interviews with offenders have convinced me that people in general are just plain easy to fool. What makes fooling us so easy is not the worst in us, it is often the best. As one rapist said,

Because people want to believe in something. They want to hope. And they want to believe. They want to, there's something inside of people that makes them want to believe the best in things and the best in others. Because the alternative is not very nice.

True enough. The alternative is not very nice.

3

Techniques of Deception

The Double Life

There are specific techniques sex offenders and other predators use to fool people. First and most important is setting up a double life. Many offenders will deliberately establish themselves as the kind of person who wouldn't do that kind of thing.

> I lived a double life. . . . I would do kind and generous things for people. I would give families money that did not have any money that was not from the church treasury, it was from my own bank accounts. I would support them in all the ways that I could. Talk to them, encourage them. I would go to nursing homes. Talk with the elderly. Pray with the elderly. I would do community service projects. Pick up litter off the side of the road. I would mow the lawns for elderly and handicapped people. Go grocery shopping for them.

The man talking was the youngest deacon in his church. It is not a surprise, really, that he rose so fast. Not many other young men in their twenties were mowing lawns, giving money to the poor, or getting up in the middle of the night to help the sick. Most were pursuing their own interests at that age. It turns out, so was he.

Sitting across from him, I wonder why he leaves me cold. He is boyish and good-looking, his smile ready and even, his eyes lively and intelligent. He has good eye contact. But something about his persona does not work. It is not the constant power-thrusting of the thug for whom life is a series of encounters that one side wins and one side loses. Nor is it the predatory delight of the psychopath who enjoys fooling people just for the sake of it and brags about it later. No, there is another note here. I settle in to listen. He is telling me that he used to choose emotionally disturbed children to victimize, kids who had histories of lying. That way, if they did disclose, no one would believe them. And they didn't. Referring to one victim, he says:

> When he did tell, and when it became a bigger issue, when I was investigated, the head of the department of my county told me, "You have nothing to worry about." He said, "We can tell from the beginning that this is all a big scheme." And it was dropped almost as quickly as it came about.
>
> I was told on twice before being incarcerated. . . . They were not believed the first two times. I had many people: counselors, church leaders, leaders of the community, to come up and stand in my defense, several times on those occasions, and it was simply just disbelief.
>
> Even the second time it was more stood out against than the first time because they thought here he goes again, this young man trying to help unfortunate children, and they're turning against him and I, I had a minister come to see and tell me, he said, "Patrick, what's going on—you'll run across it many times— people you try to help will stab you in the back," he said. "Roll with the punches, stick with it, you're doing a good job and in the end, you'll be blessed for it."

The man who will be "blessed" was eventually incarcerated for molesting a male child in his youth group. Unbeknownst to the judge or the community, he had ninety-five other victims to which he later confessed, confirmed by polygraph. All were children from his youth groups, from among the children he supervised and counseled. And he is only in his early twenties.

Absentmindedly he rubs the front of the borrowed clothes I brought him to wear in the film. The small luxury of wearing street clothes pleases him. Truly, he looks more himself in this sweater and slacks than he did in the orange prison jumpsuit. But I can visualize him even better in a suit, coming out of the service and leaning forward to clasp the hand of an elderly parishioner who would be telling him what a nice young man he is.

The charm I find strangely cold worked better in the outside world. It was not difficult to persuade people he was innocent. They were so seduced by the double life he was leading that there wasn't much persuasion to it.

Sometimes the words were not even necessary. Like I said before, they immediately rallied to my defense when I was accused of being a sexual offender. They said, "We know this young man. He has been in our community all of his life. We know his parents, his grandparents, his aunts, his uncles. This is not something that he would do. This is not something that goes along with behavior that we see him in day in and day out," and that was true because I was very careful that they did not see that behavior day in and day out. Most of my deviant behavior happened at night time and behind the scenes and away and far from my important people who could make those kinds of judgments that yes, indeed, Patrick is the kind of person who would go around molesting children.

It is here I detect a sole note of passion when he talks about the split between his real life at night and the important people who made up his day world.

But why am I uneasy here? I am used to the double life. Used to child molesters with high numbers of victims. Accustomed, even, to their choosing children who were in some way impaired.

Casting about, I go further afield. I ask him if pain and suffering is sexually arousing to him. I don't know why I ask. This man's behavior, as far as anyone knows, was manipulative and sneaky. He conned children into sexual activity, but he has no known history of torturing them or even physically striking them. But still, what does it mean that no one suspects it? No one suspected him of being a child molester either.

"Yes," he tells me easily. "In my fantasy life, definitely pain was a factor."

"But you never acted on it?" I say, surprised. It is a stupid question, and I regret it instantly. The way I phrased the question invites a "no," and I get one, several in fact.

"No, no, no," he tells me quickly. I wait for the full retraction, the "I-would-never-do-anything-like-that-it-was-only-a-fantasy," but it never comes. "The fear of leaving a mark," he says quietly, instead, "a fear of somehow leaving something that could be seen and detected and questionable kept, prevented me from doing that."

He is a sadist, although fearful of acting on it. It is at the heart, I think, of my uneasiness. There is a peculiar coldness to the sadist, even from behind the persona of the nice young man. And although I tolerate well the ingratiating charm of the child molester or the amoral delight of the psychopath or even the rage of the vindictive rapist, this peculiar coldness marks my soul.

A budding sadist posing as a minister? Not the first time. In one study, 30 percent of sadists who had killed three or more people had reputations as solid citizens,[1] and in another, sixty-five percent were middle class.[2]

But it is not just sadists who practice a double life: A double life is prevalent among all types of sex offenders. There are exceptions: offenders living in subcultures so violent or disempowered that they do not have to pretend to be less violent than they are. Like Avery, Emma's psychopathic husband (see Chapter 1), they simply intimidate or assault anyone who objects.

More often offenders establish these abusive conditions in their homes but stop short of portraying themselves to the outside world as violent. The front that offenders typically offer to the outside world is usually a "good person," someone who the community believes has a good character and who would never do such a thing. Sometimes if the molestations and rapes are occurring outside the home, they even portray the same image to their family. A man I will call Mr. Woodard tells me:

> Actually I was living a triple life. I was living one life when I'd go out with different friends, happy-go-lucky, plenty of money to spend. Everything's fine. Everything on me. Where at home with my wife I was another person. I was loving, caring, considerate. Easy to get along with. Tried to give her everything she asked for, and at work I was another totally different person. Totally real quiet, reserved. Dedicated to my work. Come in early, leave late. This type of thing. This went on for probably five or six years.

Mr. Woodard's polite, socially responsible front hid a continual string of rapes and molestations.

> Q. How many victims did you have totally?
> A. I have ninety victims total. Eighty from the ages of about four to about forty-five.
> Q. How many of these are hands-on offenses? Molestation and rape?
> A. I have approximately ninety hands-on victims. Both male and female. More female.

The persona will often shift, as it did in this case, depending on what the person in front of him wants to see. Mr. Morgan, a knife-wielding rapist of adults and children, reports:

> I lived a life of a chameleon or a salamander, changed colors with the wind. I didn't just live a double life. I lived multiple lives. Whatever life the situation called for, I lived it. If I hung around Christian people and I knew that they were Christian, then my actions and my mannerism were similar to theirs. And I adapted to whatever the situation required. If I hung around people who cursed and used vulgar language and smoked dope, then I

adapted to that situation. I could feed back to people what I thought they wanted to see and what I thought they wanted to hear.

For others, the double life is a kind of refuge from the reality of the self. A violent rapist of children tells me:

I led a double life. In the store I was an entirely different person. Maybe not so much in attitude or the way I acted, but I could be me. I could be a productive person, and I could be a decent person in the community. It was a place where I could say I'm a decent person, and when I went home I had to face this again. I'm not a decent person. I'm an indecent person. I do immoral things. . . . I loved work. I loved to stay at work because I didn't have to go back home and face my real self.

"Character" is the term we apply to the continuity we all want to see between public and private behavior. People act in accordance with their characters—or so we think. "He would never do such a thing," we say, shaking our heads. But "character" ignores the real issue of deception. Even violent predators know enough to keep their behavior in check publicly—most of them anyway. The lives they lead in public may be exemplary, almost surreal in their rectitude. Consider Mr. Raines, who says to me:

I want to describe a child molester I know very well. This man was raised by devout Christian parents. As a child he rarely missed church. Even after he became an adult, he was faithful as a church member. He was a straight A student in high school and college. He has been married and has a child of his own. He coached Little League baseball. He was a choir director at his church. He never used any illegal drugs. He never had a drink of alcohol. He was considered a clean-cut, all-American boy. Everyone seemed to like him. He was a volunteer in numerous civic community functions. He had a well-paying career job. He was considered "well-to-do" in society. But from the age of thirteen years old he sexually molested little boys. He never victimized a stranger. All of his victims were friends. . . . I know this child molester very well because he is me!

I met Mr. Raines in a prison, but he was soon out on parole. Once outside he almost immediately infiltrated a church and became, once again, director of the children's choir. I know of at least two incarcerations for child molestation subsequent to this. Still, despite this track record, I believe in my heart the next time Mr. Raines gets out of prison, he will successfully ingratiate himself in youth activities in a church once more. He will do this even though he now has at least three criminal convictions for child molestation and likely more, all of which any church could have discovered. But who will check criminal records for such an outstanding, polite, well-spoken young man? After all, volunteers are hard to come by.

Priests, of course, have had a leg up on this business of the double life because the role itself has traditionally been respected. The term "priest," like "doctor," carries a connotation of someone who is dedicated to helping others, someone who is there to provide solace and comfort. Although a double life can be practiced in any profession, it has been easier for priests to convince people they are good than it is for, say, used car salespeople or lawyers.

There are even some adolescent offenders smart enough and with enough self-control to set up a double life. Absolutely the most dangerous adolescent child molester I have ever evaluated was a fifteen-year-old boy who had anally raped every male child for whom he ever babysat. Unfortunately, he had babysat a large number of children. He was a straight A student, always neatly and appropriately dressed, always polite and helpful to the parents. He never had green hair, never had any part of his body pierced, and never drank alcohol or took drugs. Parents considered him pretty much the ideal babysitter. They didn't notice that he never hung around with other adolescents, that he always seemed anxious to spend time with younger children, and that he was particularly eager to babysit.

Sex offenders are well aware of our propensity for making assumptions about private behavior from public presentation. They use that information deliberately and carefully to set up a double life. It serves them well but doesn't do much for the rest of us.

Deception One on One

The double life is a powerful tactic: There is the pattern of socially responsible behavior in public that causes parents and others to drop their guard, to allow access to their children, and to turn a deaf ear to disclosures. But a surly and obnoxious person would have little access, no matter how proper and appropriate his public behavior was. The second tactic—the ability to charm, to be likeable, to radiate sincerity and truthfulness—is crucial to gaining access to children.

"Niceness is a decision," writer Gavin De Becker wrote in *The Gift of Fear*. It is "a strategy of social interaction; it is not a character trait."[3] There are days I want to tattoo this on my forehead. De Becker is right, but who believes him?

The man in front of me is a Southern good-ole-boy, the kind of man I grew up with and like. If anything, I have a weakness for the kind of Southern male who can "Sam Ervin" you, the Southern lawyer who wears red suspenders in court along with twenty-five-year-old cowboy boots and who turns his accent up a notch when he sees the northern expert witness coming. A "northern city slicker" on the witness stand will elicit the same kind of focused interest that a deer will in hunting season. You can have some very long days in court with men who wear red suspenders and start by telling you how smart you are and how simple and dumb they are.

I survey the man in front of me. I am not in court; I am in prison, and he is not an attorney but a sex offender, and he has bright eyes along with that slow, sweet drawl. He is a big man, slightly balding, and he has—I have to admit there is such a thing—an innocent face.

In basketball, it is not the hands you pay attention to, it is the hips. The hands fake left, right, all around, but where the hips go, the player goes. I am looking for the hips, something that will tell me what is going on here. It is always hard to figure out, especially with those hands in your face. The distracting hands are not just the Southern accent and the innocent face. In the world of lying, the "hands" are called eye contact and fidgeting.

Our culture agrees on the signs of lying. Ask any audience—as I have—how to tell if someone's lying, and it will tell you it's lack of eye contact, nervous shifting, or picking at one's clothes. This perception is so widespread I have had the fantasy that, immediately upon birth, nurses must take newborns and whisper in their ears, "Eye contact. It's a sign of truthfulness."

The problem is that sex offenders had those same nurses. If a sex offender is breathing who doesn't know to keep good eye contact when he's lying, I haven't met him yet. Eye contact is universally known to be a sign of truth-telling. People can fake eye contact; therefore, in reality, it absolutely is not a sign of truth-telling because liars will fake anything it is possible to fake—a commonsense conclusion that research confirms.[4]

My Southern good-ole-boy certainly knows eye contact is considered a sign of truthfulness. He describes his manner in getting away with close to 100 rapes of adults and children:

> The manner that I use when I was trying to convince somebody— even though I knew I was lying—I'd look them in the eye, but I wouldn't stare at them. Staring makes people uncomfortable and that tends to turn them away, so I wouldn't stare at them. But look at them in a manner that, you know, "look at this innocent face. How can you believe that I would do something like that?" It helps if you have a good command of the vocabulary where you can explain yourself in a way that is easily understood. Dress nice. Use fluent hand gestures that are not attacking in any way.
>
> It's a whole combination of things. It's not any one thing that you can do. It's a whole combination of things that your body gestures and things that, "Look, I'm telling you the truth, and I don't know what these people are trying to pull. I don't know what they're trying to prove, but I haven't done any of this. I don't know

why they're doing this. You can check my records. I've got a good record. I've never been in any trouble like this. And I don't know what's going on. I'm confused."

The truth is, the nervousness we all look for as a sign of lying can be suppressed with practice. And people do practice when their liberty and private obsessions are at stake. It is a simple point, but one I didn't fully appreciate before this round of interviews. As if reading my thoughts, he breaks off: "You don't get this, Anna, do you?" he says. "You think that when I'm asked, 'Did I do it?' that's when I lie. But I've been lying every day for the last twenty-five years."

Of course, he's right. If someone is committing sexual offenses, he has been lying since the day it began. With that kind of practice, normal signs of nervousness wear off. He becomes a "practiced liar," a category of liar that the researchers find consistently difficult to detect.[5]

But even when dealing with people who don't practice, such as college students who have volunteered for a research study of lying, most observers are not as good as they think in detecting deception. The research shows consistently that most people—even most professional groups such as police and psychologists—have no better than a chance ability to detect deception. Flipping a coin would serve as well.

If it is hard to tell when ordinary people are lying, how much harder would it be to detect the man in front of me? He is no ordinary college student participating in a research study of deception but a practiced and committed liar who knows his liberty depends on it. He is a professional, really. He has thought all of this through:

If you want to deny something, make sure you've got an element of truth in it. It sounds like it's true, and there are elements of it that are very true that can be checked out, and try to balance it where it has a little bit more element of truth than it does lie, so when it is checked out, even if the lie part of it does come out, there's more element of truth there than there is lie.

For instance, the lady that I was accused of raping, the night I said I had an affair with her. There was enough element of truth there in the fact that I did go over to her house quite regular alone and do odd things around the house because the type work I did. It was a new home, and there was a lot of kinks that needed to be worked out of the electrical system and what have you. And me making so many trips over there, and she admitting this, it was easy to check out that at least once or twice a week I would go over to her home and work on something.

And with that element of truth there, to the frequency that I went over there, it was pretty easy to convince people that it had been going on. That I had been having an affair with her for a while. Because it had been going on, I had been going over there since they moved into the home, which had been about a period of about six months.

But he was not having an affair with her. Instead he broke into the woman's home at 2:30 in the morning when her husband was not home and raped her with both her babies in the room, one of them in her arms.

He was drunk when he raped her—by her account as well as his. Still drunk when the police picked him up the next morning. Even though I think I am less naïve than most, would I ever have suspected that he spent months setting this up, that the decision to rape her was made stone-cold sober six months earlier when he started coming over to her house more often than was necessary to do the little things that needed fixing? When he was leaving his car around conspicuously for the neighbors to see during the day? Or would I have accepted it as a drunken impulse? "You don't really get this, Anna," he said to me, and it was true. But I am not the only one who doesn't get it.

His act was good enough that once he got away with stomping out of court in a huff over a previous case. He was accused by his sister of raping her and molesting her daughter on the same day. He played it as a preposterous charge. His sister, he told the court, had once accused his uncle of abuse. She was well known in the family for making up crazy charges like this. He said he wasn't going to put up with such nonsense and walked out. No one stopped him, and no one ever called him back. The charge just disappeared somehow. He admits now both accusations were true.

Such careful planning is not unusual with sex offenders. Although treatment programs routinely target impulsivity, in fact many offenders are not at all impulsive. A young musician describes to me a process of planning and careful implementation that is anything but impulsive. Once again, it is likability and charm that he wields as weapons.

When a person like myself wants to obtain access to a child, you don't just go up and get the child and sexually molest the child. There's a process of obtaining the child's friendship and, in my case, also obtaining the family's friendship and their trust. When you get their trust, that's when the child becomes vulnerable, and you can molest the child. . . .

As far as the children goes, they're kind of easy. You befriend them. You take them places. You buy them gifts. . . . Now in the process of grooming the child, you win his trust and I mean, the child has a look in his eyes—it's hard to explain—you just have to kind of know the look. You *know* when you've got that kid. You know when that kid trusts you.

In the meantime you're grooming the family. You portray yourself as a church leader or a music teacher or whatever, whatever it takes to make that family think you're OK. You show the parents that you're really interested in that kid. You just trick the family into believing you are the most trustworthy person in the world. Every one of my victims, their families just totally thought that there was nobody better to their kids than me, and they trusted me wholeheartedly with their children. . . .

Q. At church, you did not molest all the children at church. How would you choose? . . .

A. OK. . . . That's a good question. First of all you start the grooming process from day one . . . the children that you're interested in. . . . You find a child you might be attracted to. . . . For me, it might be nobody fat. It had to be a you know, a nice-looking child, wasn't fat. I had a preference maybe for blond hair, but that really didn't have a lot to do with it.

You maybe look at a kid that doesn't have a father image at home. You know, you start deducting. Well, this kid may not have a father, or a father that cares about him. Some kids have fathers but they're not there with them. . . .

Say if you've got a group of twenty-five kids, you might find nine that are appealing. Well, you're not going to get all nine of them. But just by looking, you've decided, just from the looks what nine you want. Then you start looking at their family backgrounds. You find out all you can about them. Then you find out which ones are the most accessible. Then eventually you get it down to the one you think is the easiest target, and that's the one you do.

The glint in his eye when he says this is unmistakable. I have shown a film of this man when I give talks, and from the back of a room of 250 people, the glint is still striking. No question this man is sexually attracted to little boys, but it is a hard call to say what matters to him more: the sexual contact with the children or his cleverness in fooling their parents. His cleverness does not stop at getting access; he uses it to protect himself from discovery as well.

Q. How did you keep your victims from telling?

A. Well, first of all I've won all their trust. They think I'm the greatest thing that ever lived. Their families think I'm the greatest thing that ever lived. Because I'm so nice to them and I'm so kind and so—there's just nobody better to that person than me. If it came down to, you know, if it came down to, "I have a little secret, this is our little secret," then it would come down to that, but it didn't have to usually come down to that. It's almost an unspoken understanding.

Q. Do you think any of the families ever became suspicious of you?

A. I'm sure they become suspicious, but that's where I begin my grooming on the family again. . . . If a family becomes suspicious, well, they're not really going to bring it to me, they're going to bring it to the kid first. And the kid, I've got the kid so well groomed that the kid's going to bring it to me and say, "Well, my mom asked me, you know, if you've ever tried to do anything to me or anything like that."

Well, then I begin working on the family by still being kind of nice to them but maybe backing off of that child just enough to where that parents' suspicion gets back down again. Maybe I'm not with them as much. I won't maybe have as much physical contact. I won't put my arm around the child as much. I'll do everything, whatever it takes to convince that family that there's not a problem.

This young musician admits to more than 100 child victims—I suspect he has many more than that—and out of all these, only one child told and was believed. When the last investigation broke, many of the other parents of children he molested would not even let social services or the police talk to their children. Some of the families still write to him in prison. He could *not* have been a child molester, and he most certainly never molested *their* child. After all, nobody was ever better to their child than he was.

When he's done describing all this, he tells me flatly, "child molesters are very professional at what they do, and they do a good job of it." I do not argue with him.

Now you see him; now you don't. Even after a felony conviction for child molestation, this man moves effortlessly, easily into jobs with children. He is the offender, alluded to earlier, who was able to infiltrate a church and become involved with youth activities almost immediately after being released from prison.

"Father, do you take ex-cons?" he had said meekly to a minister a few days after being released.

"Well, son, if they're truly repentant, we do."

"Oh, I am, Father. I was in Stevens Point for passing a cold check. You can check up on me if you don't believe me. And while I was there, I found the Lord, and there was this hymn I dearly loved. And I knew it would be a sign from God, whatever church was playing that hymn, that was the church for me. And Father, when I walked by your church this morning, you were playing that hymn."

Of course, the minister did not check up on him. He believed that Mr. Raines would not have suggested it had he not been telling the truth. It is an old tactic. The Boston Strangler reported that he would suggest that women call the superintendent if they doubted he was really a maintenance worker. The women took that as a sign he must be who he said he was and routinely let him in their houses without calling.[6]

Had the minister checked up on Mr. Raines, however, he would have found that his crime was child molestation, not passing a cold check. He might have been less eager then for Mr. Raines to take over the children's choir.

When the authorities eventually caught up with Mr. Raines, they found he was operating not in one church but in two. The second minister said, "Well, we thought he was sincere. You see there was this hymn that he dearly loved when he was in prison. And when he walked by our church. . . . "

I do not feel rage at Mr. Raines as I do at those who use physical violence against children. Nor do I feel the chill, the sense of a cold finger on my soul I get when talking to sadists. It is more a sense of wonder in his presence—that such people could exist.

I woke up last night worrying about an evaluation I hadn't finished. I can obsess about a bill I forgot to pay, a present I forgot to send, a thank-you note I didn't write. Most people are like me. This man's callousness rests hard on the heart. I cannot find a place for it.

But even though I don't "get it," I know what it means. Mr. Raines will give no quarter, release no hostages. He will take whatever advantage he can get. He is intent on winning, and childhood trust is his chosen battleground. We are most certainly his targets as much as our children. After all, the children, he tells me, "are easy," and Mr. Raines likes a challenge. His camouflage is expert, and he knows us far better than we know him. We have our own reasons for not wanting to see him for who he is, and he knows that too.

4

Child Molesters

Mention "child molesters" to the average audience, or even to most professional audiences, and they will immediately suggest "Colt .45 therapy" or castration. Once a cab driver in Dallas gave me his opinion: execution for a first offense.

It is a strangely comfortable answer for those who give it, and it absolves them of the harder work of thinking of something we might actually do in this country. The strangest part of this answer is that those who see child molesters as monsters seem the quickest—when their neighbor, friend, or family member is accused—to say that it is definitely a false report. After all, child molesters are perverts, creeps, and monsters, and their nice neighbor/minister/father/uncle/friend/priest is not a monster. Ergo, he is not a child molester.

Once this kind of denial locks in, no amount of evidence will change their minds. A cab driver said to a colleague of mine, "Child molestation! I know all about child molestation. My father was accused of child molestation, and the children lied—all twenty-six of them."

Even a confession by the offender will be dismissed. A long-term molester of boys tried to tell his own minister he was offending. "Someone said I was a child molester," he began tentatively.

"Well, that's the stupidest thing I've ever heard of," the minister said quickly. "You're the last person I'd believe that of." End of conversation.

But it is a misconception that child molesters are somehow different from the rest of us, outside their proclivities to molest. They can be loyal friends, good employees, and responsible members of the community in other ways. The psychiatrist Fred Berlin has noted:

People often confuse issues of traits of character with issues of sexual orientation or the type of sexual interest an individual has. People who may be compulsive pedophiles, for instance, may obey the law in other ways, may be responsible in their work, may have concern for other persons.[1]

What is different about child molesters is only this: They have sex with children. They molest them for a variety of reasons that may leave no telltale signs in their public behavior. The priest who works tirelessly for the parish may be a nice man in his everyday dealings with people, but that has nothing to do with whether he is or isn't privately a child molester.

Even angry child rapists (a minority of child molesters, to be sure) may behave normally in public. They may have a girlfriend or wife, may be well liked. No one may see the grinding anger that drives them except their victims. The child rapist below is a six-foot-tall Marlboro man with a crooked smile and a soft crinkle to his eyes. He is good-looking, and, more than that, he looks like a kind man. Not surprisingly, he has a long history of girlfriends. Indeed, with his looks and his soft and reasonable manner, he has had no difficulty attracting women. He tells me that:

First victim, I was staying with a guy. . . . His daughter had come to live with them, and I was living with them at that time. And I was angry. She had done a lot of things, like I'll just give you an example. The very first time I had a Zippo lighter, and I'd get it hot and just play with it. . . . She came in one day, and she was playing with it and got it hot, and I was laying on the couch and I was asleep. She brought it over to me and put it on my forehead and burned my forehead, which made me very angry. I didn't say much to her then. But that afternoon, or that night, when her mother was at work, I raped her that night. Which it was anally at the time. And it went on for quite some time before I, I called it an accident because she wasn't able to endure intercourse. . . . And it ripped her.

In fact, he tore her anus through to her vagina, and the eight-year-old child was injured so badly she was hospitalized. He was incarcerated for that offense and later served a second incarceration for a separate offense. In between there were numerous offenses he was reported for but for which he was never charged. He shrugs and tells me:

> People, in general, they're going to think what they want to think. And that's just basically all there is to it. If they want to think bad of you they're going to think bad of you. If they hear something bad of you they're going to believe it, and if they don't, they don't. In the business I was in, you know, this guy works around children all the time. If he was molesting children, there's no way you couldn't get caught.

It was perhaps an exaggeration for him to say he worked around children all the time. He was night manager at a grocery store, and there were probably fewer children in the store at night than during the day. Still, despite enough anger and callousness to rip an eight-year-old from vagina to anus, he appeared perfectly normal to those who worked with him. I do not believe anyone in the world, including myself, could have picked him out as a child molester.

But even if you and I couldn't see it in casual conversation, the anger and the intimidation were there—in his case, only for children. And he used it right in front of us and got away with it. He tells me how he handled disclosures by the children:

> Basically if you stay calm and look whoever it is in the eye, and especially if the mother of the victim or the victim is there, if the victim is anywhere that you can look at her and make her nervous or him, whichever one it might be, then the more nervous that you make them, the more it makes them seem like they're lying. If they're around. Most of the time they're not.
>
> Q. How do you make them nervous?
>
> A. By staring at them. You know, it's like, I'm going to get you. I'm just, it's just basically, you know, just that kind of look. Like

you've had it. To a child that's, you traumatize them just by looking at them.

Court is just another opportunity for intimidation in his view.

If we went to the court and we both had been in the courtroom at
the same time, then I could have made her nervous enough to
make her lie or make her stumble to make people think she was
lying. . . . It's really just a simple look to a child is traumatizing. If
you believe it or not, it really is. Especially if the adult is molesting the child.

He does not have to convince me that offenders will try to intimidate
witnesses in court. I was on the witness stand once against a man who
had raped and murdered a nine-year-old neighbor child who came to his
door on Halloween night. He was scheduled for release, and I was testifying that he was still dangerous and should be civilly committed, a case
that was lost. I'm not sure it would have been lost had the jury been looking at him rather than me. He glared at me throughout my testimony as
though he would take my throat out with a spoon. A part of me wanted
to interrupt my testimony and just point to his sullen, rage-filled face.

I could not do so, of course, and unfortunately almost everybody in
the courtroom was looking at me. The spectators had no choice: They
were sitting, as usual, behind the defendant. There was, however, a single correctional administrator who was sitting far enough on the side to
see the defendant, and she was looking at him while I spoke. She was
so taken aback by his obvious hostility and his attempt to intimidate me
that she came to talk to me about it afterward.

If it was sobering for me to testify with a predator glaring at me,
imagine what it is like for a child. It is easier than you think for offenders to intimidate witnesses in open court and get away with it. Now you
see it; now you don't. Child molesters, angry rapists, predators of all
sorts only show the face they want you to see, when they want you to
see it. And sometimes, they give you the message they want you to
have, even though no one around you sees a thing.

Making Sense of Child Molestation:
Blind Allies and Hidden Bias

Why do men—and some women—molest children? It makes no sense to the rest of us. Our collective difficulty in believing someone we know would molest a child is partly because of our difficulty in understanding why anybody would do such a thing. Most adults are simply not sexually attracted to children. When an adult is in an amorous mood, a child is a nuisance at best. "What would a child have to do to be sexually attractive to you?" an instructor asked a class rhetorically.

"Grow up," one man replied.

Most of us feel that way. Sex with children strikes us as deeply reprehensible and utterly unappealing. If that's how most people feel, why do child molesters risk jail for something the rest of us wouldn't do if it were legal?

In the past one hundred years, psychology has twisted itself into pretzels developing theories to answer this question. Few of these theories have any research at all behind them, and many of them are little more than excuses and rationalizations for child molestation. I am not talking now about Freud's failure to accept the victim accounts given by his patients and his turning them into "Oedipal fantasies" to avoid ostracism by his peers. That has been too well documented to deserve further comment.[2] Nor am I talking about cases where memory of abuse was lost and then recovered, although there is considerable evidence that this can occur.[3]

What is actually more perplexing in the history of psychology is the attitude toward cases in which it was known and acknowledged that the abuse took place. In the early part of the century, psychoanalytic writers maintained steadfastly that sexual abuse was the fault of the child, not the adult, that it occurred because aggressive children "seduced" innocent men. Dr. Karl Abraham, for example, wrote an article entitled "The Experiencing of Sexual Traumas as a Form of Sexual Activity" in which he declared that "in a great number of cases the trauma was desired by the child unconsciously, and we have to recognize it as a form of infantile sexual activity."[4] His reasoning was that "in all of them the trauma could have been prevented. The children could have called for help, run away or offered resistance instead of yielding to the seduction."[5]

It is bewildering, of course, that Abraham would not recognize the existence of psychological coercion or just plain submission to adult authority, but after all, it was 1907. It is more puzzling that he would not apply the same logic to the offender who, after all, could have called for help, run away, or offered resistance. Yet Abraham did not call his article "The *Inflicting* of Sexual Traumas as a Form of Sexual Activity."

What is truly astonishing, however, is his response to a case of violent assault in which the child did call for help, run away, and offer resistance. In fact, she resisted so much she escaped. It was the case of a nine-year-old girl who was enticed into the woods by a neighbor who Abraham admits "attempted to rape her."[6] The child fought off her attacker. Rather than admit that responsibility for this attack rested solely with the attacker, Abraham states that the child

> Had allowed herself to be seduced. She had followed the neighbor into the woods and allowed him to go a long way in carrying out his purpose before she freed herself from him and ran off. It is not to be wondered that this child kept the occurrence secret.[7]

It is most surprising that Abraham could ignore the difference in strength between a nine-year-old girl and an adult male. In his view, no matter what the circumstances, all sexual assaults on children occur because children have "an abnormal desire for obtaining sexual pleasure and, in consequence of this, undergo sexual traumas."[8] Women assault victims fared no better in his hands. They were labeled "hysterics" and were described as

> Those interesting people to whom something is always happening. Female hysterics in particular are constantly meeting with adventures. They are molested in the public street, outrageous sexual assaults are made on them, etc. It is part of their nature that they must expose themselves to external traumatic influences. There is a need in them to appear to be constantly exposed to vi-

olence. In this we recognize a general psychological characteristic of women in an exaggerated form.[9]

If Abraham's views were not echoed elsewhere, he would be simply a historical oddity. On the contrary, his views were widely shared within the psychoanalytic community. For more than fifty years, from the first quarter of the twentieth century onward, there was a significant school in psychology that held that sexual assault victims were responsible for their own victimization.[10]

The psychiatrist Lauretta Bender was a strong supporter of this point of view and wrote in 1937 that such children derive "fundamental satisfaction from the relationship" and "do not completely deserve the cloak of innocence with which they have been endowed by moralists, social reformers and legislators."[11] As proof, she offered her observation that the children were "unusually charming and attractive"[12] and asked the reader to consider that the child was "the actual seducer rather than the one seduced."[13]

The concept of "participating" or "collaborative" victim was developed.[14] In many of these writings, a participating victim was anyone who knew the offender prior to the attack and/or was assaulted more than once. However, this rule wasn't ironclad. The researcher John Gagnon characterized 12 percent of his sample of children assaulted by total strangers as "collaborative," whatever that term means to him.[15]

Incest victims seem particularly singled out for this blaming of the victims. Dr. Irving Weiner wrote that the "absence of any complaints on the part of the daughters indicates that these girls were not merely helpless victims of their fathers' needs but were gratified by the relationship, if not . . . active initiators of it."[16]

Of course, many victims did complain. Nonetheless, Weiner dismisses such reports by saying that "it is quite likely that many incestuous daughters avoid guilt feelings by denying their enjoyment of the sexual experience."[17] It is not at all clear what victims could have done to convince Weiner of their innocence. In his writings, we find that whether victims endured silently or complained loudly, they were nonetheless deemed to have been "gratified" by the incest.

A basic tenet of science is that if the facts don't support the theory, the theory should give way. It often simply does not happen. Sometimes the facts are twisted to fit the theory or if that fails, they are simply ignored. For example, Atolay Yorukoglu and John Kemph described two children who were victims of incest with a parent.[18] Between them, the two children had the following symptoms: setting fires, vandalism, stealing, aggressive behavior, sexual abuse of boys, anxiety, exhibitionism, social withdrawal, and suicidal ideation. They were kept in residential care because they were too aggressive to be maintained in a foster home. Nonetheless, the authors titled the article "Children Not Severely Damaged by Incest with a Parent" and described the children as "not seriously affected."[19] Dr. Mary de Young wondered if the children would have agreed.[20]

The most extreme view in this area was that of Matilde W. Rascovsky and A. Rascovsky, who declared that incest was actually good for the child. "The actual consummation of the incestuous relation . . . diminishes the subject's chance of psychosis and allows better adjustment to the external world."[21] It is not clear what "facts" that statement was based on, but this view was shared by at least some writers. In 1979, a West Virginia social work professor announced that "incest may be a positive experience or at worst, neutral and dull."[22]

Putting aside for a moment the absurdity of such claims, what is particularly puzzling is that the adult offender was effectively erased from these descriptions as though he had no responsibility—indeed as though he wasn't even there. When offenders are mentioned, their responsibility for their own behavior, their harmfulness and aggressiveness, are described in terms that are strikingly benign.

"Gentle, fond of children and benevolent" was the way Virkunnen described the pedophile.[23] He was a "timid person, usually without adult contact, childish and immature."[24] Drs. Eugene Revitch and Rosalie Weiss called such offenders "harmless individuals and their victims . . . aggressive and seductive children."[25] These authors complained that a group of children "*exploited*" a pedophile "through accepting his gifts and money" (italics mine).[26]

This blaming of children for child sexual abuse began to fade for a time in the 1970s and 1980s, although it has never died out entirely and is currently making a comeback. Witness, for instance, the legal defense filed by Cardinal Bernard F. Law in Boston in 2002, claiming that "negligence" by a six-year-old boy and his parents contributed to the fact that the child was sexually abused by a priest.[27] One wonders what kind of negligence he's talking about on the child's part.

Note too that a California judge, also in 2002, sentenced a thirty-three-year-old teacher to probation instead of prison after she was found guilty of having sex with a fifteen-year-old boy. The judge stated that "the relationship may have been a way for the boy to 'satisfy his sexual needs.'"[28]

To the extent that making the victim responsible for abuse did wane, however, its waning brought with it a shift of responsibility, not to the offender, initially, but to the nonoffending spouse and the family instead. Blaming the mother has actually been embedded in the incest literature for some time, although it began to achieve much greater prominence as blaming the child began to fade. The incest offender was said to be "placed in the position of compensating the oral frustrations inflicted by the mother."[29] Irving Kaufman et al. wrote that incest was the child's response to abandonment by the mother,[30] whereas Lillian Gordon declared that the child committed incest as revenge against the mother for pre-Oedipal frustrations.[31]

Where was the father? Captain Noel Lustig and his colleagues considered the father little more than a "vehicle" for "unconscious homosexual strivings in the mother."[32] They wrote of the father's "psychological passivity" while calling the mothers the "cornerstone of the pathological family system."[33]

Mothers supposedly gave permission for the incest, unconsciously if not consciously. Some authors felt that the percentage of mothers who knew about the incest approached 80 to 90 percent.[34] Blair and Rita Justice disagreed, insisting that *every* mother colluded with the abuse in some way.[35]

In the late 1970s, a child sexual abuse treatment was developed by Hank Giarretto in San Jose, California, that became nationally famous and served as a model for the development of many other treatment programs. The statement of philosophy for the program declared that

"Incestuous behavior is one of the many symptoms of a dysfunctional family."[36] Giarretto proudly published figures that showed the percentage of mothers who felt responsible for the incest rose from 0 percent at intake to 50 percent at termination. This was considered success.

I attended a training at that treatment program in the 1980s. The culpability of the family, including the victim, was stressed so much that I finally raised my hand.

"If I was an offender in this program and I reoffended," I began, "I'd just say, 'Guess the family's not doing too well.' How are you going to hold people responsible for this if you tell them it's not their fault, it's the family's fault?" There was a lot of scrambling but no answer given that made sense to me.

This line of reasoning sometimes went to absurd lengths (if you don't think it was there already). Yvonne Tormes, for example, described a group of incest offenders, some of whom had been extremely violent.[37] They had burned children with hot irons, locked a mother in a closet while abusing the child, and broken a radio over a mother's head. One would think the offenders might have some responsibility for their behavior in these cases, but Tormes wrote that the cause of the abuse was "the mother's failure to protect her child."[38]

Today, the notion that the family is responsible for incest is far more alive than the notion that children are responsible for seducing grown men. There are still numerous treatment programs that use family therapy to treat incest. Whereas some use family therapy responsibly, as an adjunct to offender treatment, others state openly that they consider incest to be caused by family dysfunction and that treatment should address the family problems, not the offender's proclivity to offend.

Of course, considering the family the source of the abuse inevitably means reducing the culpability of the offender. In 1989 Clinicians Terry Trepper and Mary Jo Barrett described their method of doing family therapy with offenders.[39] They recommended telling the family, "The incestuous abuse may indicate that your family loved each other too much."[40] Child sexual abuse is thus redefined simply as "loving too much." Could it be a little confusing for a child to have incest labeled as "love"?

A colleague of mine described an adolescent victim's reaction to treatment such as this. He was in individual therapy with my colleague as well as family therapy with another therapist. One day he said to my colleague, "Is there some rule in family therapy that you can't point the finger at anybody?"

"Sort of," my friend acknowledged.

"Because sometimes," he went on, "I think that therapist forgets who is the fucker and who is the fuckee." Point well taken.

The history of psychology in the past one hundred years has been filled with theories that deny sexual abuse occurs, that discount the responsibility of the offender, that blame the mother and/or child when it does occur, and that minimize the impact. It constitutes a sorry chapter in the history of psychology, but it is not only shameful, it is also puzzling. Hostility toward child victims and adult women leaks through this literature like poison. What accounts for the kind of foam-at-the-mouth hostility expressed by Professor of Law Ralph Slovenko in 1971, when he railed against the laws that held offenders responsible for sex with a child and quoted a 1923 judge's ruling with which he evidently agreed?

This wretched girl was young in years but old in sin and shame. A number of callow youths, of otherwise blameless lives as far as this record shows, fell under her seductive influence. . . . She was a mere "cistern for foul toads to know and gender in." Why should the boys, misled by her, be sacrificed?[41]

He added that "the male offender in the case of statutory rape has no special pathology; the girl is usually more in need of psychiatric care or other attention."[42]

If these views seem dated and extreme to you, you might want to consider Judith Levine's new book, *Harmful to Minors*, or an article by Bruce Rind et al. on the impact of child sexual abuse, or a recent paper by Professor Harris Mirkin,[43] all three of which have received enormous press—much of it positive—and all of whom minimize child sexual abuse and its impact. Levine, in fact, wants to lower the age of consent to twelve. Rind and Mirkin both question whether sexual abuse harms the child, and Rind, in fact, would like us to quit calling it abuse.

These views bear looking at more closely. Levine's book, particularly, is troubling: The case she makes is flawed by numerous inaccuracies and misstatements of fact. Levine claims there is simply no large-scale problem of child sexual abuse. She argues that most normal men are attracted to adolescents, and therefore the attraction isn't deviant at all. She minimizes or even ignores the fact that some men are attracted to children far younger than adolescence. It is not clear, she contends, that there is any such thing as a pedophile,[44] and to prove her point, she cites the true fact that some men who are attracted to children are also attracted to adults. According to her, therefore, they are not pedophiles.

However, whether someone is attracted to adults is irrelevant to whether or not they are a pedophile. The diagnostic manual of the American Psychiatric Association states that pedophiles are adults who are sexually attracted to prepubescent children, and they may or may not be attracted to other adults as well.[45] As someone who has interviewed a number of men who have raped infants as young as five months of age, men who have sexually abused preschoolers repeatedly, men who have targeted children under the age of ten, and men who *admit* to being sexually attracted to them (some of them obsessively so), I can only wonder why Levine would make this claim.

What would she say, for example, to the three brothers I interviewed last week who were molested by a priest when they were children. One of them remembers vividly the last time the priest molested him. The priest was fondling the boy's nude genitals when he noticed the boy had begun to sprout his first pubic hair. The priest stopped immediately.

"What's this?" he demanded.

"It's hair," the child said. "It's been there."

"I never noticed it," the priest said, and got up immediately. That was the last time he molested that child. But he continued to molest his younger brothers.

But it is not just Levine's denial that pedophiles exist that makes this book troubling. She believes that even if pedophiles do exist, they can be "cured."[46] That is certainly news to me, and it will be news, I sus-pect, to all who treat offenders. It will be news as well to the Associa-tion for the Treatment of Sexual Abusers (ATSA), the largest profes-sional organization on the treatment of sex offenders in the world. ATSA states plainly on their website that, "although many, if not most, sexual abusers are treatable, there is no known 'cure'. Management of sexually abusive behavior is a life-long task for some sexual abusers."[47]

The best estimates today, based on a analysis of forty-three studies of treatment and reoffense rates, is that current methods of cognitive-behavioral treatment can reduce sexual offending by close to half in the relatively short run.[48] The impact of treatment can be summed up in an odds ratio of .60. Not every offender would reoffend without treatment, of course, but for those who would, treatment can make a difference. Out of every one hundred offenders who would have reoffended, sixty would still reoffend with treatment. This reduction in reoffending is ac-tually heartening. Being able to reduce reoffense rates by nearly 50 per-cent certainly makes treatment worthwhile in my book. The forty out of one hundred offenders who would not molest again after treatment translates into numerous children who will be spared abuse if offend-ers get proper treatment. Certainly treatment is more efficacious today than it's ever been in the past.[49]

But sixty out of one hundred sex offenders would still reoffend after the most effective treatment available today, and that means we are a long way from "curing" pedophilia or rape. Note also these results were for the short run. No one really knows the impact of treatment in the long run.

No one in my field today even speaks of a "cure," any more than al-cohol and drug counselors speak of a cure for alcoholism or drug ad-diction. Given all that, I looked with interest for the source of Levine's optimism, but she offered no research, no support whatsoever for her notion that pedophilia is curable, except her own interpretation of re-search on reoffense rates.

Contrary to politicians' claims, the recidivism rates of child sex of-fenders are among the lowest in the criminal population. Analyses of thousands of subjects in hundreds of studies in the United States and Canada found that about 13 percent of sex offenders are rearrested, compared with 74 percent of all prisoners.[50]

But her comments about 13 percent reoffense rates are only accurate to a point, and the point is a big one. The major meta-analysis she cites only studied reoffense rates for all sex offenders (treated and untreated combined) in the first four to five years after release.[51] The implication Levine makes that these are lifetime reoffense rates is wrong.

Research on long-term reoffense rates finds considerably higher rates.[52] Dr. Robert Prentky, for example, found that the long-term reoffense rate for rapists was 39 percent and for out-of-home child molesters, 52 percent.[53] Conservative estimates from across studies show that it is likely that no fewer than 40 percent of child molesters and rapists reoffend in the long run. These are average reoffense rates, and they refer to *detected* offenses. Obviously, we don't catch people for everything they do. In fact, the rate of detection of sexual offenses looks quite low, as noted earlier. But even ignoring the issue of underreporting, close to half of child molesters are likely to reoffend in the long run, most certainly not 13 percent as Levine claims.

Certain subgroups of sex offenders are known to have even higher rates of reoffending. The Canadian researcher Karl Hanson found that those offenders who were never married, had boy victims, and had previous offenses demonstrated a detected reoffense rate of 77 percent in the long run.[54] Any group with a detected rate of reoffense that high means that virtually all offenders in those groups are likely to reoffend, given what we know about undetected offenses.

Did Levine not know all this? Did she really misread the research so completely that she believed that 13 percent was the lifetime reoffense rate of sex offenders, or did she simply feel it would not help her case to state accurate figures? Her case states that pedophilia doesn't really exist, that even if it does, it can be easily cured, and that—not to worry—child molesters don't reoffend very often, anyway.

But what is very troubling about this book is that Levine goes far beyond inaccurate figures, naïve assessments, and a poor fund of information; she goes on to give advice to parents and legislators, specifically that we should lower the age of consent to twelve. In Levine's world, there is no problem with twelve-year-olds having sex. And it is not just sex per se that Levine encourages for young teens, it is specifically sex with older men.

> Teens often seek out sex with older people, and they do so for understandable reasons: an older person makes them feel sexy and grown up, protected and special; often the sex is better than it would be with a peer who has as little skill as they do. For some teens, a romance with an older person can feel more like salvation than victimization.[55]

Despite the rosy picture that Levine paints of sex between young adolescents and adult men, read her book carefully, and you will discover she cites research that found negative consequences to adult/child sex. Girls in relationships with older men often agree not to use a condom; they also frequently drop out of school and/or cut off ties with friends and families. These same girls later on often speak negatively of these early relationships and "regretfully of their choices."[56] Levine hastens to inform us, however, that the same thing might have happened with younger lovers. But the same thing wouldn't have happened with no lover.

Other studies have found similar results. A study by the National Campaign to End Teen Pregnancy found that two-thirds of sexually active twelve- to seventeen-year-olds wished they had waited until they were older: 72 percent of the girls and 55 percent of the boys.[57]Although Levine tells us repeatedly to listen to children when they say they want to have sex with adults, here she tells us not to listen. The teens don't know their own minds, she informs us. Their regrets can be traced to societal attitudes. "Teens get the message that the sex they are having is wrong, and whenever they have it, at whatever age, it is too early."[58] Maybe, but maybe they were too young, just like they said.

Apparently, we should not listen to our children, to what happens to their lives when they get involved in sex too early, to what happens when they become involved with older men. We should not listen to their regrets or their health problems or their young pregnancies. Instead, we should only listen to what twelve-year-olds want in the heat of the moment.

Levine is not alone today in minimizing the effects of child sexual abuse and in trying to redefine it. In 1998, Rind et al. published a meta-analysis of studies that looked at the impact of child sexual abuse on college samples.[59] Despite the fact that the samples they used were all from college populations, they use their findings to make statements on child sexual abuse in the larger population, although later they claimed they were only saying it was "relevant," not representative or generalizable.[60]

Their conclusions were—although victims were more maladjusted in seventeen of eighteen categories of maladjustment—that the maladjustment was slight and due to family dysfunction, not child sexual abuse. When family dysfunction was controlled statistically, the difference in maladjustment supposedly disappeared.

Boys in particular, they felt, were not affected by child sexual abuse. Although Rind et al. admitted that that impact could be separated from wrongfulness, they nonetheless recommended dropping the word "abuse" and calling sex between adults and children simply "adult-child" and "adult-adolescent" sex instead. The term "abuse" would only be used if "a young person felt that he or she did not willingly participate in the encounter *and* if he or she experienced negative reactions to it" (italics mine).[61]

Presumably, then, forcible rape of a child would not be considered abuse even if the child did not "consent," provided the child later said the abuse had made her or him stronger (a positive reaction) or the child minimized the impact as adults have repeatedly been shown to do with traumatic events of all sorts.[62]

Likewise, the seduction or manipulation of a child into sexual activity would not be considered "abuse" by definition, even if trickery, bribery, or conning was used and even if the child had a severe reaction. According to Rind et al., unless there is violence, the child "consented." Rind makes no distinction for children under twelve in these definitions. Presumably, a four-year-old—or even an infant—is able, in their view, to give "consent" because consent is simply defined as the absence of overt violence.

The study kicked up a storm in two very different quarters. First of all, experts in the field were surprised, to say the least—I among them. I had read the literature on the impact of child sexual abuse carefully for some time, particularly so for a book I did on treatment of victims.[63] I initially planned on reading *all* the literature on the sequelae of child sexual abuse, but that grandiose plan faded as I read for months on end without being able to tap into all the research. At the end of several months, however, I was convinced of one thing. Child sexual abuse was like getting bitten by a rattlesnake: Some kids recovered completely, and some didn't, but it wasn't good for anybody.

But if scholars familiar with the literature were surprised by the study, others were outraged. Dr. Laura came across the study, and nine months after its publication told 18 million listeners on March 22, 1999, that it was "garbage research with a dangerous statement at the end."[64] She added that she thought the study might be used to normalize pedophilia and to change the legal system, which is certainly exactly how certain groups have used it.[65]

The publicity resulting from Dr. Laura's radio address was so great that even Congress got involved. In July of 1999, they passed a resolution condemning the study, a first to be sure. Unfortunately, for many academics, the issue then became a question of academic freedom. In defense of the study, academics pointed to the fact that it had survived peer review, supposedly a rigorous process.

But had it? It was later revealed that it had been rejected by the first set of peer reviewers, and the authors were told the study was so flawed it should not be resubmitted. However, after a change of editors, Rind et al. tried again. This time at least one reviewer also turned the study down. Because the others have not come forward, it remains unclear as to who actually recommended the study for publication, if anybody.[66]

The study has been repeatedly criticized on methodological grounds. Apparently some who read it think the original reviewers got it right. Critics have charged that Rind et al. excluded relevant outcomes, included studies with primarily noncontact offenses (such as exhibitionism), used inappropriate statistics, and generalized their results inappropriately, among a host of other flaws.[67]

Rind et al. have put up a vigorous defense.[68] As a key element in that defense, they have attacked everyone in sight for bias. They have called their critics "religious and moralistic zealots."[69] They have portrayed themselves as representing "science" and their critics as representing "moralistic psychiatry," "politics," and "orthodoxy."[70] They have even compared themselves in workshop flyers to Galileo and Darwin.[71] They have accused everyone else of bias, but nowhere have they mentioned their own.

But the fact is that Rind at al. were pro-pedophilia long before their meta-analysis was published. Take, for example, their articles in *Paidika: The Journal of Pedophilia*. *Paidika* is not your typical objective academic journal. In fact, *Paidika* does not pretend to be objective at all. It is published in the Netherlands, where the age of consent has been lowered to twelve, and its purpose was summed up in its first issue as follows:

> The starting point of *Paidika* is necessarily our consciousness of ourselves as paedophilies. . . . We intend to demonstrate that paedophilia has been, and remains, a legitimate and productive part of the totality of human experience.[72]

I came across this journal some time ago, when I discovered that a psychologist who frequently testified for the defense in child sexual abuse cases, Ralph Underwager, had given an interview to this journal in which he said pedophilia was a "responsible" choice, called it, "God's will," and stated it was about "closeness and intimacy." The cover of that issue had a drawing of a nude adolescent boy on it.[73]

Both Rind and his colleague Bauserman had published articles in *Paidika* long before their meta-analysis appeared, Bauserman arguing that pedophilia has traditionally provided boys with positive role models, and Rind commenting favorably on a book that attacked the "child abuse industry."[74] After the meta-analysis appeared, they were keynote speakers for a conference on pedophilia in the Netherlands, sponsored by an organization whose head, Reverend H. Visser, is a long-term advocate for pedophilia.[75]

In addition to his writing for *Paidika*, Bauserman also wrote a spirited defense of Theo Sandfort's work in another article. Sandfort had contacted pedophiles who then selected from their current victims those he could interview. Sandfort spoke with the children, then reported that they experienced the relationships and the sexual contacts positively. Despite the fact that the activity was illegal in the Netherlands at the time (where the study took place) and despite the fact that many of the parents did not know their children were being abused, Sandfort did not inform the authorities or their parents but colluded with the pedophiles' secrecy and deception.[76] Understandably, Sandfort's work has been attacked on both methodological and ethical grounds.[77] Bauserman's article attacked Sandfort's critics and justified Sandfort's methods and his conclusions. Bauserman was barely out of college at the time and was about to enter graduate school. His meta-analysis was eight years away.

It does not appear that these are objective, neutral scientists here doing a let-the-chips-fall-where-they-may study. At least two of the three original authors were writing positively about sex between men and boys long before their meta-analysis "discovered" there was "little harm" attached.

But their own biases aside, the real question is whether the study is any good. The statistical arguments fly back and forth, and for any reader who would like to follow them, I refer you to the citations above. But two things are clear: The first is that their findings are truly an outlier. As Stephanie Dallam points out, other meta-analyses have obtained very different results.[78] In addition, a series of studies controlling for family dysfunction have found that when you remove the impact of other social variables, including family dysfunction, the negative impact of sexual abuse remains.[79]

The second fact that's clear is that, one more time, the offender has disappeared. In Rind and his colleagues' view, kids are either forced into sexual acts through violence or they "consent." The underlying assumption is that children and adolescents are equal matches for adults. Presumably either adult pedophiles are *not* trying to manipulate and con children for sex, or it is a "buyer beware" situation in which the kids can and should fend for themselves.

But the former is absurd, and the latter is unfair. It is surely not just my own observations that offenders manipulate children. Lucy Berliner and Jon Conte interviewed twenty-three child victims of child sexual abuse, aged ten to eighteen years.[80] Half of the children described being given special favors, money, or clothes. The process of moving from normal physical affection (for example, hugs) to overt sexual acts was subtle and accompanied by rationalizations. The children were told that the behavior was acceptable, for example, that it was a way to show love or that it was a form of sex education. Most of the children had developed strong emotional ties to the offender. According to Berliner and Conte, more than half said they "loved him, liked him, needed or depended on him."[81] Then, too, almost all of the children were threatened with harm either to obtain their "consent" or to prevent them from telling. The threats were various: cutting fingers off, cutting the child's throat, killing the child, or abandoning them.

Sex offenders themselves will tell you that they use techniques deliberately to seduce and entice. Jon Conte, Steven Wolf, and Tim Smith found that offenders believed they were skilled in identifying vulnerable children.[82] They quote from their sample of twenty sex offenders as saying:

I would probably pick the one who appeared more needy, the child hanging back from others or feeling picked on by brothers and sisters.[83]

I would find a child who doesn't have a happy home life, because it would be easier for me to gain their friendship.[84]

Look for a kid who is easy to manipulate. They will go along with anything you say.[85]

Choose children who have been unloved. Try to be nice to them until they trust you very much and give you the impression that they will participate with you willingly. Use love as bait. . . . Give her the illusion that she is free to go with it or not. Tell her she is special. Choose a kid who has been abused. Your victim will think that this time is not as bad.[86]

Other research agrees. British researchers Michele Elliott, Kerin Browne, and Jennifer Kilcoyne found in a sample of ninety-one offenders that nearly one-half said they chose children who "seemed to lack confidence or had low self esteem."[87] They manipulated the child's affection through bribes, gifts, and games.

This process of manipulation is based on important differences in maturity levels, without which the manipulation wouldn't work. The child is at a disadvantage here: He or she has no idea of the offender's intentions, no way to know that the affection expressed isn't genuine, and no recognition of the techniques used to manipulate him or her. Most writers who defend pedophilia—Rind, Bauserman, and Levine, for example—simply pretend this kind of manipulation does not occur and that children and adolescents are equal partners with adults in sexual activities.

However, Harris Mirkin takes a different view. An associate professor at Kansas State University, he wrote an article that compared the "oppression" of pedophiles to the oppression of women and homosexuals. Evidently aware of the extent to which pedophiles manipulate adolescents, he simply justified it.

Pubsecents and adolescents are usually thought of as hard to control and attempts to mold their behavior and initiate them into legal and enjoyable adult activities are considered valuable. However, in the sexual area these assumptions are reversed. It is asserted that they are easily controlled, and they are conceptualized as little children who have no sexual desire of their own and can only be passive victims. According to the dominant formulas the youths are always seduced. They are never considered partners or initiators or willing participants even if they are hustlers.

It is only legitimate to coerce pubescents and teens not to have sex. It is argued that they cannot give consent, that they cannot enjoy sex even if they think that they do, and that they suffer physical and psychological harm, even if they are not aware of it. . . . [88]

In other words, why not manipulate adolescents into having sex, much as we put pressure on kids to do their homework or brush their teeth?

The old gang would be proud—Abraham, Virkunnen, Revitch and Weiss, Bender and Blau, Lukianowicz, Henderson—everyone who minimized child sexual abuse, denied the role of the offender, and put all the responsibility on the children for "participating." Child sexual abuse is once again "infantile sexual acting out." Besides, sex between men and children—these new advocates tell us—doesn't do any harm, anyway, and we're just being moralistic by calling it "abuse."

Even the old invective is back. This time it is less often attacking the children or even the mothers, although some have done so. This time the invective is mostly for those who evaluate or treat abused children or advocate for them. In Rind's world we are "religious and moralistic zealots" attacking the modern equivalents of Galileo and Darwin.

In Levine's world, Andrew Vachss, the attorney and mystery writer, becomes a "sex-thriller writer,"[89] although if there is anything Vachss doesn't do, it's describe sex with children in any way that makes it "thrilling." Joyanna Silberg, a former president of the International Society for the Study of Dissociation, is described as "discredited," although she's never even had a board complaint filed against her, and her reputation is solid among her peers.[90] And when referring to Adam Walsh, a six-year-old boy whose head was found floating in a canal, Levine writes that his case "helped spur the creation of the National Center for Missing and Exploited Children and (some say) the career of his father,"[91] a comment that is as callous as it is offensive.

The hostility to children and those who advocate for them continues. The attempt to minimize and deny the reality and impact of child sexual abuse is alive and kicking.

Men Who Are Sexually Attracted to Children

Unfortunately, despite Levine's contention, pedophiles exist, as do men who molest children for other reasons. The reasons they molest them are far simpler than complicated (and conveniently unprovable) theories of "unconscious homosexual strivings in the mother."[92] Sex offenders do not molest because they are magically bewitched by aggressive and seductive children, nor do they because they are "compensating the oral frustrations inflicted by the mother,"[93] as quoted in Lustig et al. It is not due to alcohol or stress in their lives. Nor is it because they are simply "in love" and the age difference irrelevant. The age difference is always relevant. In fact, it is the point. A sizable proportion molest children simply because they are sexually attracted to that age group. They have what is most often termed a "deviant arousal pattern."

The labels for this group have differed throughout the history of the field, but the group's existence has always been recognized whenever an actual analysis of the offenders has been done. Any division of child molesters into subgroups has always found a set that is sexually attracted to children. The researcher Paul Gebhard called them "patterned" as opposed to "incidental" offenders.[94] Swanson spoke of "individuals to whom the child represents the sexual object of choice" as opposed to "those on the other end of the continuum where the choice of an immature sexual object is virtually a matter of convenience or coincidence."[95] Kurt Freund described offenders who were primarily attracted to children versus those who used the child as a surrogate for an adult partner.[96] Nicholas Groth divided offenders into "regressed" and "fixated,"[97] whereas Richard Lanyon used the terms "preference" versus "situational."[98] Hilary Eldridge described them as "continuous" versus "discontinuous" offenders.[99]

All of these terms describe similar concepts. What has been clear for thirty-five years or more is that some offenders are fixated in their sexual interests. Their sexual attraction to children is sometimes exclusive and sometimes in conjunction with an attraction to adults as well.

It is a particularly vexing group because, for one thing, we don't have a clue how and why a sexual attraction to children develops (although that doesn't stop people from proposing theories about it that are presented as absolute fact). But if we don't understand the origins, we certainly know something about the patterns it produces. A deviant arousal pattern appears to begin early and to be as rigid as normal hetero- or homosexual preferences, and as resistant to change. In early

PREDATORS

adolescence, when most of us are finding peers attractive, the dreams of preferential child molesters are filled with much younger children. They start masturbating to these fantasies of sex with children, and for some of them it becomes their exclusive form of sexual fantasy. The child molester below describes how early he began fantasizing about children and how consuming those fantasies became.

Q. How old were you when you began to have sexual fantasies about children?
A. About 13 or 14.
Q. When you masturbated in the three months prior to the commission of your offenses, how often would you say during masturbation you had sexual fantasies involving children?
A. All the time.

This is not an unusual answer for a child molester. I ask another about his sexual interest pattern:

Q. Before you got into actual involvement, sexual involvement with these boys, was there any masturbation that was going on with fantasy about having sex with them?
A. All the time. That's a constant thing with me. It's something I'm still working on right now. I have to get, I have to calm that down. I believe if I can get a hold of that, I'll do a lot better.
Q. How much of the time do you fantasize about boys?
A. I'd say about half the day. It's when I'm not doing anything.

This is, of course, the reason that prison does nothing to change the sexual interest pattern of such offenders. They spend their lives thinking, fantasizing, masturbating, planning, and molesting children. Prison stops the molesting most of the time (although I know of cases—and have even testified in one—in which an inmate molested a child in the visiting room). But surely, prison at least slows the actual molesting down. By itself, however, prison does nothing about the fantasy and the planning. The obsession is maintained by constant masturbation to fantasies of children. The inmate emerges from incarceration at least as deviant as he went in.

In some ways, the group that molests children because they are sexually attracted to them makes some sense. At least we have a motive. But whereas some child molesters are sexually attracted to children, there is no credible evidence that all offenders have a deviant arousal pattern, and there is considerable evidence that some do not.

But what would account for someone risking jail, their livelihood, their relationships with family and friends, and most certainly the condemnation of the community to have sex with children, if they are not even sexually attracted to them?

Problems and Their Relationship to Child Sexual Abuse

People are meaning makers. When we don't know the answer, mostly we just make it up. Experts seem to choke on the words "I don't know" and give answers that defy logic and lack evidence to avoid admitting ignorance. There is no paucity of "answers" to the question of why sex offenders without a deviant arousal pattern molest children. Alcohol, family stress, job stress, marital problems, financial problems, abuse as a child—all have been suggested repeatedly as "causing" child sexual abuse. But these are only theories, and there are significant problems with each of them.

Imagine yourself all alone on a Friday night after a long week. Let's say you are out of town at a meeting. You're far from home and feeling lonely, and you have a relationship or marriage that isn't going well. Having sat in your room for the previous three evenings, you find yourself in a pleasant bar with a glass of wine and a colleague of the appropriate gender for you. After two glasses, you notice how attractive your colleague is. Strange, you hadn't thought much about it before. After the third glass, you decide your colleague is really quite witty. Just about everything he or she says seems to be extremely funny and charming.

What happens next would never happen to you, personally, of course. But in the course of human history, it has happened that in such circumstances, certain individuals' judgment has gone downhill. In fact, some people's judgment has taken an Olympic bobsled run downhill, shattering all known records. But at that moment of vulnerability in the bar, if a three-year-old boy walked in, would he look any better to you as a possible sex partner than he does right now?

Alcohol releases inhibitions and decreases judgment concerning sexual interests the person already has. It will not create a sexual interest the person otherwise lacks. Likewise, all of us face stress without resorting to child molestation. It is striking that in twenty years of dealing with child molestation, the stresses offenders cite seem so ordinary: financial problems, marital problems, job problems. Child molestation seems highly unlikely to relieve that stress in the rest of us.

Although we may not entirely understand why, it is still clear that some men who molest children do not have a deviant arousal pattern. Certainly, we can identify other reasons some of them molest. Psychopaths will sometimes use anyone to gratify their sexual needs: children, animals, adults. Also, some with the inclination to molest seem worse under conditions of stress, but many molest when things are going well. Clearly, loneliness plays a role for some.[100] A significant percentage of child molesters do not seem to know how to connect with adults, and they alleviate their loneliness through children whom they find more trusting and accepting. But why sexualize it?

Finally, the most common answer in the literature has been that molesters were sexually victimized themselves as children. It has become a truism in the field. But is it so?

Are Child Molesters Really Just Victims Themselves?

"All victims are offenders," one professional challenged me at a conference, "and all offenders are victims. How does your work address that?"

My work doesn't address that because I don't believe there's any evidence for that assertion. Obviously, not all victims are offenders, but also it is likely that most offenders weren't victims. The studies that find a high proportion of child molesters who were victims of child sexual abuse themselves are almost always based on self-report, and even there, study results differ dramatically. Studies show the number of child molesters who were themselves molested as children ranges from 22 percent in some studies to 82 percent in others.[101]

But in any case, offender self-reports have dubious validity, especially when the offender's self-interest is at stake. The only rule for deception in sex offenders I have ever found is this: If it is in the offender's best interests to lie, and if he can do it and not get caught, he will lie.

Being victimized as a child has become a ready excuse for perpetrating child molestation. The offender who claims he himself was victimized gets seen as less of a "monster" than one who wasn't a victim, and he gains much more empathy and support. It is hard to trust self-reports of sex offenders about abuse in their past when such reports are in their best interest.

Only a few studies on this topic have used objective measures, and they have found very different results.[102] Jan Hindman knows all too well that people who have lied for decades about their offending would lie to her about being victimized as a child, so she compared the reports of abuse by child molesters who were not being polygraphed on their answers with a later group who was informed that they would have to take a polygraph after the interview. The group that was being polygraphed was also given immunity from prosecution for crimes previously unknown in order to take away one of the many reasons that offenders lie.[103]

This study is not about how good the polygraph is—although it appears to be highly accurate[104] and better than people are at detecting deception in any case. Rather, this study is about how good the offenders thought the polygraph was because the answers of the group who *was going to* take the polygraph turned out to be very different from the group who wasn't going.

In a series of three studies, the offenders who claimed they were abused as a child were 67 percent, 65 percent, and 61 percent without the threat of a polygraph. With polygraph (and conditional immunity), the offenders who claimed they were abused as children were 29 percent, 32 percent, and 30 percent, respectively. The polygraph groups reported approximately half the amount of victimization as children as the nonpolygraph groups did.

Nonetheless, the notion that most offenders were victims has spread throughout the field of sexual abuse and is strangely comforting for most professionals. For one thing, it gives meaning to the behavior of offenders and at the same time allows people to feel badly for them. I remember a cartoon in which a man is lying in the gutter, badly beaten. Two social workers stand over him, and one says to the other, "The man who did this really needs help." If offenders are just victims, then no one has to face the reality of malevolence, the fact that there are people out there who prey on others for reasons we simply don't understand.

Even people who know better collude with this stance. A professional I know is fond of telling audiences, "The victim you don't treat today is an offender tomorrow." I called her up.

"That isn't true," I said. "The studies don't back that up," and I rattled on about polygraph and the dubiousness of offender self-report.

"It doesn't matter," she replied. "I can't get them to care about what happens to victims if I don't say that."

I thought about it when I hung up. Basically she was saying that scaring half the molested children in the United States into thinking they will be child molesters when they grow up is justified by political expediency.

But I am not being honest here. My problem with her approach is not primarily that it frightens people. Many true things frighten people, and lying about them doesn't help. If the statement were true, I would not suppress the information. My problem is that it isn't true. This woman is frightening victims about something that isn't even true. She doesn't think it matters whether it's true or not and considers me a goody two-shoes, an obsessive academic. She sees herself as someone who sees the larger picture.

She could be right about a lot of this. Probably I am a goody two-shoes—certainly, an obsessive academic. Maybe she does see the larger picture. But a couple of decades of swimming in deception has left me holding onto the true things, clutching them in my little paws, turning them over and over. A true thing has a different ring, a different energy about it. It leaves little wake and does not disturb the complex interweaving all around it the way a lie does.

These lies: They glitter, spin, and undulate like lures trailing through clear water, but always, always there is a hook embedded somewhere under all those feathers. Call me an obsessive academic. I'll check every figure in this book before I release it. It's not a moral stand. It's just a need for one true thing.

So What's the Answer?
Why Do Offenders Molest Children?

We only know this much. There is a subgroup of child molesters who molest children simply because they are sexually attracted to them. There are others who molest because they are antisocial or even psychopathic and simply feel entitled. There are still others who use children for the intimacy they are too timid or impaired to obtain from adults. And there are others who molest for reasons we don't understand at all.

But make no mistake, whether men molest because of sexual preference or for other reasons, their compulsiveness can be extraordinary. Take, for example, a minister who had sexually abused his grandchildren. He had no criminal record of any sort outside the sexual charges and, in fact, had lived a responsible life in every other way. When he was caught, he admitted the offenses and made no excuses. He pled guilty and was imprisoned; he told me he was glad to be in jail because he thought it could make up, in some small way, for what he had done. I asked him how he had justified the abuse to himself while it was going on, how he had put aside the conscience that was evident elsewhere in his life. He responded:

I didn't suspend my conscience. I carried it right into the action with me. I think in my own personal view this is part of a compulsive pattern. You do things, you don't always justify the action, but you carry the consequences of the action into the action, and you do it despite or in spite of the known consequences.

I suppose that being a devout religious person, if I had believed with all of my mind and heart that the earth was going to open up and swallow me up in hell, I would have went ahead and done it anyway.

I remember distinctly my reaction when he said this. The hair stood up on the back of my neck. I understood for the first time what we were up against. If a man who truly believes in hell would be willing to go there in exchange for the chance to molest a child, this problem had a persistence and a compulsiveness that few outside the drug addiction world could appreciate.

Whatever the reasons people develop such a fixation, it tends to be chronic and resistant to change. The people who have such patterns are not a small number, more like an invisible army that cannot be recognized on the street. Certainly, some of them are unemployed, take drugs, and fulfill the stereotype of the street criminal. But there are others considerably more successful in life, and they may be equally goal-oriented and driven in pursuit of children: the college professor who traveled to the Philippines to buy children from poverty-stricken parents, the Olympic-level kayaking coach who threatened to ruin the kayaking career of any student who resisted, the teacher who used questionnaires to identify the children with low self-esteem and then molested them, the minister who researched families to find out who didn't have a father, the priest who held a boy underwater when he tried to resist.

These men—and they are usually men for reasons we also don't understand—are part of our communities, part of our network of friends, worse yet, sometimes part of our families. Some of them are doctors and lawyers, and some are academics who publish studies. No one has all the answers about how to stop them, nor even why all of them do what they do. But at least we should have the decency as a people to stop making excuses for them.

Female Sex Offenders

By all accounts, female child molesters are less common than male ones, but they do exist. How common they are depends on where you look. For example, if you look at reports that come into child protection agencies, about 3 to 5 percent of them involve female offenders.[105] If you look at who's serving time in prison, the figures go down. A Canadian study found that less than 1 percent of sex offenders serving two years or more were female.[106] That certainly fits with my experience. It is far rarer for female sex offenders to be prosecuted than male, and far more difficult to get convictions. The average person does not seem to want to believe that women, particularly the child's own mother, could do such a thing. Once, when I was presenting on female sex offenders, the first question from the audience was, "How do you stay sane?" No one has ever asked me that when I present on male sex offenders.

Female sex offenders appear to be different than male offenders in some important ways. There are three basic types of female offenders that keep appearing in the research literature,[107] and they do not match exactly the typology of male sex offenders. First, one of the largest groups is a group that molests children under the age of six, primarily their own. Many of these mothers seem to be fused with their children and unable to function as a maternal figure. For example, an adult survivor cited by Bobbie Rosencrans described her mother as follows:

> She wanted me to love her like her own mother did when she was little and sick. It makes me nauseated to think about it. She used me to maintain her own sick pleasure. I was mother, father, husband, sister, lover and friend to her when I needed a mother.[108]

The really bad news is that many of these molesters of young children have sadistic tendencies. In Jacque Saradjian's study, nine of the fourteen offenders in her sample admitted to enjoying hurting the child. That some of these women are truly sadistic is evidenced by the descriptions of some of their adult offspring.

> My mother threatened to burn my hair/me if I did not comply. I was given beer to drink. I was beaten and there were threats I would be burned if I wasn't quiet. Sometimes I was slightly burned on the butt with lit cigarettes. I learned not to cry and to stop screaming.[109]

Another survivor stated that "the more I hurt the faster she'd come."[110]

Secondly, there is a teacher/lover group that primarily molests teenagers. This is not a group of teachers or adult women who are eighteen or twenty and are involved with seventeen-year-olds. There was, on average, a sixteen-year age gap between offender and victim in this study. Thus, these are a group of adult women, generally in their thirties, who pretty much double the age of their victims.[111] These women do not, in general, act sadistically. How could they, given that they do not have the same degree of power and control over their victims that a mother does over a young child? The victims simply would not comply. The women, instead, romanticize their involvement with the teens and tend to deflect the responsibility for it onto their victims.

The last group has no parallel in the world of male sex offenders. It is a group of women who are initially coerced into having sex with a child by a male partner. Their initial motivations are generally to please the male or, at the least, to avoid abandonment by him. However, as time progresses, some research indicates that many of these women begin to enjoy the sex with children and eventually molest them on their own.[112]

Regardless of the type of offender, women offenders are capable of the same severity of sexual abuse as male offenders are. Nor does the lack of a penis stop them from penetrating a child. A study listed all the objects that had been inserted into children's vaginas and rectums by female offenders. They were as follows:

Enema equipment, sticks, candles, vibrators, pencils, keys, hairbrushes, hairbrush handles, light bulbs, soapy wash cloths, wooden spoons, various fruits and vegetables, knives, scissors, lit cigarettes, sock darning tools, surgical knives, hair rollers, religious medals, vacuum cleaner parts, goldfish.[113]

There may be fewer female sex offenders than male ones, but it would be a serious mistake to think they don't exist or to underestimate the harm they do. Male or female, child molesters are difficult to spot. Their interest in children may be compulsive, but it is almost always well hidden. If they make mistakes, they are usually small ones. Now you see them; now you don't.

I am standing in the gym at a children's sock hop. The noise is deafening. Two hundred children are running, hopping, sliding, dancing, and whirling, all the while simultaneously shrieking at the top of their lungs. There is such a thing as a perpetual motion machine, and it is called childhood. The yelling children and the blaring rock music make me hunger for the quiet and the solace of my little fireplace and the book I left behind. Because neither of my children has given a backward glance since they headed into the fray, I begin to wonder why I'm here. The mother of my daughter's best friend had invited both of my children to come with her, but I had been reluctant to give them up. I work so much that time with my children is precious.

"This is spending time with your kids?" I think. I feel foolish and out of place. I don't see anyone I know. I trudge grumpily over to check every twenty minutes or so just to keep track of my kids. It is a neurotic impulse, I think. What could happen in such a public place?

I find my daughter. At age six, she is dancing happily with her best friend and another girl and the other girl's father, a man I don't know. I wave and turn away.

Twenty minutes later I look for her again. She is still dancing with the same group. It crosses my mind that this is a little unusual. In a setting like this, her attention span is normally measured in nanoseconds, not in forty-minute blocks. Usually she has to see everybody, explore every corner of the gym. Why is she still there?

Twenty minutes later the same group is still dancing. I am uneasy now; this is simply not her pattern. I walk over and touch her arm and turn her to dance with me. Instantly the man grabs her arm and pulls her back, right out of my hands. I take her arm again, give him a look that would freeze blood, and yell, "I am her mother" over the blaring rock music. He backs off. My daughter and I and her best friend go off to dance together.

After that I keep an eye on her—and him. He ignores his own daughter, but when he thinks I am not looking, he finds mine and her best friend in a long line of kids waiting to go under a limbo pole. He looks around, then picks both of them up and throws them in the air, all the time smiling and laughing and focusing on them intently. I step up, and he slips off.

A few days later I call on my daughter's teacher. I was uncomfortable, I tell her. No other father in the room was hanging around other people's children in that way. It was inappropriate, and if that man comes to school, I don't want him alone with my daughter. "Funny you should say that," she says. "He showed up for a field trip the other day. He spent so much time with another child that I thought he was that child's parent and sent a note home to the wrong family."

I go home and tell my nanny. Someone's going to call, and it won't be him. Likely it will be the child, perhaps the mom. They're going to invite my daughter over to play. Just be ready because she isn't going.

"What do I say?" my nanny asks, panicked. "I don't know what to say."

I stare at her incredulously. "Tell them she's sick," I say evenly. "Tell them she was abducted by aliens. Tell them she's pulling the wings off flies or doing quadratic equations. I don't care what you tell them. But she is never going."

Within a week, the call comes.

I tell the parents of my daughter's best friend because she was targeted too. Their daughter doesn't go either—for a while. But time and social norms wear her parents down. "What could we say?" they ask me. "It was during the day. He wasn't home. I don't think he'd do anything during the day with the sitter there, do you?"

Maybe he won't, I think. Maybe he isn't even a child molester. Maybe I am wrong about this. But if he is, he will not hesitate to come home early from work, dismiss the sitter, and take a little girl's trusting face in his hands and tell her he will teach her a new game.

I don't know what to say to these parents. In their heart of hearts they believe what they want to believe. He is middle-class, wears a suit, goes to work every day, pays his bills, takes his family on vacation, and seems like a nice person. He is a "nice" man in their world, and niceness, they believe—they want badly to believe—is a character trait, not a decision. They are afraid of strangers. I am afraid of him.

5

Rapists

The statistics for rape tell a very odd story. Women are least safe at home and least safe with friends, acquaintances, and family. Statistically speaking, women are better off with strangers and being anywhere but our homes, at least as long as we stay away from streets and parking garages. The best thing we can do to protect ourselves is to grow older.

As noted in Chapter 1, somewhere between 12.7 percent and 24 percent of U.S. women have been raped, depending on the study.[1] According to Bureau of Justice statistics, approximately one-half of the victims of rape or attempted rape are attacked by a friend or acquaintance, and overall 62 percent are assaulted by someone they know, adding together friends, acquaintances, intimates, and family members.[2] Only about one-third are victimized by a stranger. Youth provides no immunity: The highest risk age group is sixteen to nineteen.[3] More than one-half of sexual assaults take place in someone's home, either the victim's or a friend's, relative's, or neighbor's. The most dangerous place to be outside the home is on the street.

Only about approximately 5 percent of all rapists ever spend a day in jail, and fewer still spend any significant time there. For example, in 1991 there were approximately 700,000 rapes of adult women in this country as reported in general population studies that ask women about their experiences of sexual assault.[4] Rapes of adults are actually only about a third of the rapes that occur in this country each year. In the same year, the National Women's Study reported 1.4 million rapes of children (when rape is defined as penetration).

Even if the rapist is caught, it takes time for these cases to come to trial—time for the offenses to be investigated, and time for them to reach court dockets. Therefore, we can begin to look at what happened to these cases by looking at the year 1992, rather than 1991 when the offenses were committed. In 1992 a total of 120,000 sex crimes of any sort was reported to the police. Of those, the number of offenders who were actually charged, tried, and convicted and who then spent at least one year in prison was 7,500 or less than one-half of 1 percent of the actual number of cases that had been reported to researchers. Sexual crime does indeed pay.

The rapists I have spoken with represent only a minority of rapists. Date rapists are rarely reported and even more rarely prosecuted. The men I talk to—the ones sent to prison—have almost always victimized a stranger or, at most, an acquaintance. They are a subset of rapists, to be sure, but an important one because stranger rapists are particularly likely to reoffend.[5] Also, although most of us at least believe we have some control over whom we pick as friends, all of us are vulnerable to a stranger with a knife.

But who are these men? And what kind of thinking makes it possible for someone to put a knife at a stranger's throat? What motivates them? Surely not just sex when it can be obtained by picking up someone in a bar or simply by buying it.

It turns out that there is considerable diversity among rapists, some of whom are motivated by a taste for violent sex, others by a desire to vent rage. Still others are just plain criminals who burglarize a home for the VCR but consider it a bonus if a woman is home alone.[6] They all share thinking patterns the rest of us consider distorted; they share too a willingness to use brutality to meet their goals.

Opportunistic Rapists

Some rapists are simply criminals who take sex because the opportunity arises in the midst of another crime. Consider Mr. Carlyle below:

> In my case I think it was more or less the availability. . . . I was doing a lot of burglary, stealing stereo equipment and all that stuff. Somewhere back here I was thinking what if someone's

home one of these times, what am I going to do? And this time somebody was home. It happened to be a female. Okay. So the thought was grab her. So I grabbed her. We wrestled around and I'm thinking, "Okay, I'll just tie this woman up and I'll go about my business and go on."

So as I drug her back towards the bedroom and removed her from the room because I had, my face was covered. I wanted to get this off my head so I can go on and do what I was going to do and get out of the place.

Somewhere during the over-powering I guess the feeling of "Here I am in total control of this person," overpowering, I don't know. I got sexually turned on and that's when I raped the woman. . . . It came out. It was like regurgitating. It just exploded out of me.

Q. (another offender in group) Was she attractive or was she ugly or what? If she had been repulsive to you, you wouldn't have raped her?

A. I don't even—truthfully I can't remember what this woman looks like. I haven't the slightest idea whether she's ugly, fat, or skinny. It just happened.

It always seems to amaze victims that rapists don't always recognize them in court. The crime is very personal to the victims; after all, their bodies were invaded—how could he not even recognize them? It always seems to amaze rapists that victims expect they will be recognized and that they take the attacks personally.

The man quoted above is your garden variety antisocial criminal. He doesn't care who the victim is, not even what she looks like, any more than he cares whose home he's burglarizing. He's in love with his own sense of power, and he's in search of a thrill. He's burglarizing homes because he likes to, because he finds it exciting. He doesn't need the money to survive, although in his case the money will be helpful in supporting his drug habit. He goes on to describe his motivation in burglarizing:

Q. Why were you burglarizing homes?
A. Money at the time. It's a source of easy income.

Q. You didn't have a job?

A. Yeah, I had a job. I was greedy. I could get away with bur-glary. You know, I'd done it, and we got away with it, and I kept doing it. It was my addiction.

There is a thrill when they enter someone's home that both rapists and burglars report. The following exchange is between Mr. Carlyle, the opportunistic rapist above, and Mr. Hodges, a rapist who does not commit other crimes but is a compulsive rapist (discussed below) rather than an opportunistic one. Despite their differences, they find a common thrill in home invasion.

Hodges: Did you ever get this feeling like, you know, you're going to break into a house, and it's dark and everything like that, and you find one little window or door or whatever where you can make that lock move and open and smell the air, how the air was different inside the house than it was outside the house, and just get a feeling of exhilaration when you first could just by going in whatever way you went in. . . .

Carlyle: Really, I can't say I did that. It was more the adrenaline got me. You know, the first initial step in the house. I'm in. Yeah, okay.

Hodges: Excitement, rush.

Carlyle: Yeah. It's dark or not dark. You're creeping around the corner real slow. It's eerie. It's almost a scary feeling that's going on inside you because you don't know what's around the next cor-ner. . . . Robbery, that's sexually stimulating to a guy. It's different. Running in front of a train is sexually stimulating to a degree. It gets you high. It's a high, man, that you just got to experience.

Compulsive Rapists

In addition to opportunistic rapists, there are rapists who assault to vent anger, and still others who have a primarily erotic motivation.[7] Some of the anger rapists have a pervasive, grinding rage that comes out not only in sexual attacks on women but also in physical assaults on men: They may get in barroom fights or punch out a supervisor at work. Other anger rapists, however, are just plain misogynistic. They don't attack men but reserve their hostility and aggression for women. Women are all "deceitful bitches" who deserve whatever they get. The erotically motivated rapists, on the other hand, are attracted by sex, but it is specifically violent sex that draws them.

Whatever the subdivisions, compulsive rapists do not commit rape primarily in the course of other crimes and merely because the opportunity is there. They create the opportunity because for them rape is the main event. Below are the words of a compulsive rapist with both erotic and anger elements combined. He had been peeping at women through windows for years, standing outside and masturbating. Below he describes the first time he entered the window and raped a woman.

I wanted that excitement, you know. There's this one situation where this woman had fallen asleep on the couch, and the T.V. was on but the shows have gone off. There was just fuzz, and she had on a very little negligee, and there was a very beautiful woman like Playboy and, you know, I'm looking in there, and lots of times it's a hurried, rush situation. I'm just going to catch a glimpse; let's get off here. But this is, I've got all night. She's fallen asleep, and so my fantasies were allowed to go wild, and I wanted more.

The rapist, Mr. Hodges, is telling this story in a treatment group that I am filming for a training video. The group therapist is sitting with the group, and there are also two cameramen in the room. I am off to the side with the director, watching the group. Mr. Hodges tells the story softly, hypnotically, and the group grows very still listening to him. I am the only woman in the room, and as I look around, I realize that all the men—cameramen and director included—seem to have glazed eyes. The image of a beautiful woman lying on the couch in a negligee speaks to all of them. Then Mr. Hodges continues:

I wanted some excitement, and there was some urgency there, and there was a lot of feeling, and there was some anger there, and I wanted to take a cigarette—I smoked cigarettes—and drop a cigarette in on her. Do something. Get some feeling there. Get something going.

At this point, both cameramen and the director visibly recoil. Their fantasies, wherever they were going, did not include lighted cigarettes. The director is close enough to me that I can see him blink rapidly. He puts his hands on his earphones and turns to me with an appalled look on his face. I just shrug. In the meantime, none of the offenders in the group so much as raises an eyebrow. Mr. Hodges, certainly, is unaware there is anything unusual about what he was saying. He goes on:

I think sexual drive was involved in feeling a lot of this, but there's definitely some anger coming out there, you know, and something that wants to complete this, this fantasy, this act, this whole thing, to get more to it, to get this excitement thing, you know.

So I'm going to go inside. I'll just go inside. I didn't have a mask. I didn't have gloves. I didn't have a weapon. I didn't have a plan like I'm going to do sexual intercourse, anal intercourse, oral intercourse. You know, I didn't have any plan. You know, I had these fantasies about having sex with her, you know, about sexual intercourse, but I didn't have it all put together in some plan.

I just had all this energy, and I just went to another window and opened it and went in and told her, woke her up. . . . I turned off the T.V., woke her up, and I said, "I'm just going to have sex with you."

She's going, "What do you want?" and starting to scream, you know. And I'm being real nice. You know, "I'm just going to have sex with you," like. And then she says, "Well, no." And then I grabbed her by the throat, and I said, "I'm going to rape you," and she realized the anger and violence, that the possibility was there, and then she said, "All right. Just don't hurt my child." See her child was sleeping in the other room, and that was like, I never intended to hurt your child, but I know I could manipulate you with that, and that was like information stored.

The woman began to cry and continued to cry while he raped her. Hearing this, another offender in the group asked:

Q. Was rage on your mind? When you wanted her to perform oral sex, I felt just now when you said that, that she started crying, I felt a whole lot of rage. I did. I think I would have been, if I wanted it, I wanted it and damn her crying, she was going to do it.

A. Yeah, I didn't quit because she was crying. I quit because it would be over for me, and I wanted it to last.

In this excerpt, we see the anger, the erotic component, and the callousness that accompany this type of rapist.

Distorted Thinking

If you hear no regret from the men above, it's because they have none. Not because they necessarily are psychopaths, people without a conscience, although Mr. Hodges may be a psychopath based on his overall pattern of behavior. But there are different ways to commit crimes and not regret them, and being a psychopath is only one of them.

It is also possible to avoid regret by simply rationalizing the crime. Human beings have an extraordinary ability to rationalize any sort of extreme behavior. Mr. Carlyle believes that everyone is out for number one, that there is no difference between him and anyone else, except perhaps in his boldness and his success in burglary and rape. In fact, he justifies rape by claiming it is not as bad as what some other men do to women.

With me, I've never struck a woman. I've never hit one, and it's kind of weird, I don't even believe in it. It's repulsive to me that guys can beat up women. It bothers me greatly. I've had friends who burglarized homes that had a woman home, and they nearly beat the woman half to death. I've never done that. And like I said, at the time when I raped, I was kind of thinking, well, hey, this isn't as bad as me beating her up.

This is Mr. Carlyle's claim and his excuse for the rape. But make no mistake, it does not necessarily mean that he's never beaten up a woman. To be sure of that, one would have to talk to former girlfriends, wives, and so forth. The excuses offenders use to themselves and to others are not always literally true. If confronted, for example, with a previous domestic violence report, Mr. Carlyle might easily say, well, that wasn't really a *beating*. He just pushed her around a little, and she deserved it for getting in his face. Nonetheless, true or not, the belief that he's never really beaten up a woman will make him feel better about the rape.

Of course, the psychopathic rapist has little need for such elaborate justifications. Mr. Hodges, who thinks very much like a psychopath, has an answer to how he justified the rape. The answer is simply that he wanted to do it.

Q. (from therapist) What did you say to yourself?
A. I need this. You know, I need to get off. I need some sex. I need a release. I need some relief. . . . I can't control myself. I need this, and once I do this I'll be okay. I mean it's like, let me just get this out of the way, and then I can go on with my life or with whatever I wanted to do, and it was exciting, very, very exciting, secretive. It had an allure to it. It was very powerful.

What you hear in that statement is entitlement, the belief that whatever this man wants, he should have, with no thought or concern for the wishes or welfare of others. It is a personality trait that is found in pure form in psychopaths, but it is found to some extent in many other criminals and even in some individuals with personality disorders but who don't commit criminal acts.

Mr. Morgan, the man below, groomed or seduced children and adolescents into sex. If they resisted, he simply raped them, usually with a weapon to subdue them. He feels he is entitled to sex from anyone he chooses.

> My thinking about victims that I was raping was that they were there for me to do with whatever I wanted to. They were nothing more than an object for me to have sexual gratification.
>
> I had no empathy. Didn't care. Nothing for them unless they were satisfying sexual urges that I had, rape urges that I had, and I didn't have anything for them. I thought that some of the thinking errors that I had was that I deserved this. I deserved to be treated nice. I deserved what I want. They have no right to tell me "no" when they do it all the time with everybody else. They haven't, their job is to please me and do what I tell them, and they're going to do what I tell them. Women are there for pleasure, and they're going to give me mine.

The Fantasy and the Act

The cornerstones of rape are distorted thinking and rape fantasies. These fantasies play an enormous role in the development of compulsive rapists. This does not mean that every man who has a rape fantasy will someday turn into a rapist. The rape fantasies that rapists have are distinguished from the occasional rape fantasies of nonoffending men by their prevalence, their obsessiveness, and their importance to the rapist. There are many rapists for whom the fantasies are more important than the actual rapes. It may literally be true that in some cases the rapes are committed to provide fuel for the fantasies rather than the other way around. Consider the relationship between rape and fantasy in Mr. Hodges's case.

> You know, I would think about, manufacture this beautiful woman in my mind to have sex with, and I would portray myself as a good lover, you know, a stud or, you know, have two or three orgasms and made her have an orgasm even though she was being raped.

You know, there was this little scene, fantasy that I played out in my mind, and when I committed rape, the fantasy did not live up. I mean the rape did not live up to the fantasy . . . but the rape was part of the next fantasy.

The fantasy wasn't all the same thing, like the same picture of a woman and the same sexual acts. It was different acts. It was different situations. But the rape became part of the next fantasy, you know, and in my mind—and these pictures are so vivid and so clear that I had, and these fantasies are so strong, and now I still have trouble with them. They come to me when I'm asleep, going to sleep at night. Before I go to sleep, I have them, but I don't dwell on them. See, there's the key. You know, they'll come into my mind, and I have never been able to stop them, but when they do come, I don't dwell on them.

Anyway, I would think about the rape and how I didn't do this or that, and part of the new fantasy is, you know, well, I'm going to do this or that. You know, take the old rape, put in some new parts, and I've got a new, fresh fantasy that is like the pot of gold at the end of the rainbow, kind of.

Q. (Different offender in group, very softly) Perfect.

A. Right. The perfect rape. This is what's going to make it work. This is what's going to be exciting, or this is what I need to have— that total fulfillment or that total excitement.

This emphasis on the importance of fantasies runs like a trail through the tangled forest of rapist cognition. Often these fantasies start very early and continue for years before the assaults themselves begin. Mr. Morgan began by molesting other children in his extended family. When the children wanted to stop, he didn't, and the first rape fantasies began.

The violent fantasies of rape for me began about twelve. The reason was because the individuals that I was sexually experimenting with began to realize, that hey, we were related, this is wrong, and they quit. And the ones that I was manipulating, raping, buying them gifts, and grooming, they began to realize, and they started to want to stop.

Well, I didn't want to stop. So I had to think of another way to get what I wanted, and I began to think of scaring victims into allowing me to rape them. And I began to have fantasies of using knives, and ice picks and things of this nature, to rape.

Mr. Morgan began to act out his fantasies, and eventually he raped not only relatives but strangers as well. Who the victim was mattered little to him.

It really doesn't matter who the victim is. If I can't get access to females, fourteen to sixteen, then I will settle for whatever is available at the opportunity when I'm ready to act out. I would take whatever is available.

Mr. Morgan was thirty at the time of this interview, with a long track record of violent behavior behind him, mostly toward teenage girls. His current conviction was for raping a seventeen-year-old relative, and he had been incarcerated for the past eleven years. Although he had not had access to victims for the entire eleven years, the fantasies had not dimmed. Still, they had changed.

When I was on the street, the age ranges that I masturbated to were around thirteen to seventeen. But as I came in prison, the ages started dropping off from sixteen down to twelve down to eleven, and then the fantasies increased to where they didn't have any pubic hair and things of that nature.

So I could see the degree that it's changed in eleven years. They have also switched from young females to young males. Wanting to rape young males, ages seven to nine.

The fact that his fantasies changed over time is not unusual. Sometimes the sex or age of the victim will change, and for some rapists, the degree of violence will escalate. The rapist below, whom I will call Mr.

Carron, abducted a woman from a convenience store in the middle of the day. He quietly put a gun to her back, told her to smile, and simply walked her out of the convenience store. No one knew a crime had taken place. Certainly, no one even knew this young man was at risk to commit a crime because no one knew the obsessiveness and the violence of his fantasy life.

> At first my fantasies were of consensual sex when I was masturbating. When I first started out. And they stopped to where I was reading pornography. I was thinking while watching this pornography, women, the way they posed in this pornography, women liked it rough. Women wanted it rougher. And I would get rougher with my victims, and I got more excited by that.
>
> And I continued that. And that grew for me. And to the point where around the age of fourteen I had fantasies having a large house and having the basement full of women locked up in chains. At first it was one woman, then more, then later on as the years progressed, it was more and more. And it became more and more deviant. Whenever I, I had redheads, blonds, brunettes, I could pick any victim I wanted. I'd have them all stored down there.

You Can't Incarcerate Fantasies

Steel bars and guard towers stop people but not fantasies. The men in the section above were all incarcerated, but their fantasies could not be. I am not so foolish as to suggest prisons are unnecessary—they keep offenders off the streets for a period of time. But it is a myth that prison alone will "teach the offender a lesson" and stop him from reoffending. Mr. Morgan, the rapist whose age range for victims was dropping as his fantasies escalated, tells us:

> To me, warehousing somebody for twelve or thirteen years in a penal system does nothing, without treatment, does no more than add to his deviancy. In my opinion, it just, it's an accomplice.

You're an accomplice to his crime. He's fantasizing. He gets three meals a day. He gets to fantasize all he wants to about what he wants to do, and when he gets out, he's going to carry that out. Because as a man thinks, he does.

Likewise, Mr. Carron, the man who abducted the woman from the convenience store, found prison did not interfere with his ability to develop newer and better fantasies. In fact, he used prison to reflect on the mistakes he made in the first crime that caused him to get caught.

For the first five years that I was locked up, I masturbated to a lot of rape fantasies. I knew why I had went wrong, and once they let me out, I was going to do it right . . . For me not to get caught, I'd have to plan my crimes out a lot more. In detail. I thought I had planned this one out. I had got so wrapped up in the adrenaline rush that I forgot certain aspects. I left my car parked in front of a warehouse where I had taken my victim. If I had moved my car, the police would never have come to check. They were doing a routine check and caught me.

He plans on correcting those mistakes next time.

Rape and child molestation are somewhat different from each other, not only in their choice of victim and the type of behavior, but also in the motivations that push them. It seems that a disordered arousal pattern—in other words, a sexual attraction to children—underlies many compulsive child molesters, although justifying and excuse-making surely play a role. But for rape, it is "stinking thinking": Hostile attitudes to women, a sense of entitlement, callous indifference to others, and self-serving excuses play a leading role. And it is fantasy, mental rehearsal with masturbation, that leads the way.

Once I was interviewing a rapist in prison. He was a young, healthy, good-looking man, and before he spoke there was no clue in his face or demeanor that he was someone with an incredibly lengthy record of assaults. His latest crime was as simple as it was effective. He ran his car into the back of a woman's car on an isolated road. She thought it was an accident—as he intended her to—and she stopped the car to exchange insurance information.

When she opened the door of the car, he dragged her from the car and beat her severely before raping her and leaving. The photos that were taken of the victim forty-eight hours later were so grisly that the judge, I'm told, was visibly affected, and so was this man's sentence. With a long and violent history behind him, and many previous convictions, he was sentenced as a "habitual offender" and received a term of 150 years. It was, admittedly, a stiff sentence, but one he had worked hard at earning.

At the end of the interview, he threw his hands up and said to me, "A hundred and fifty years? For a beating and a blow job?" He looked at me incredulously as though he had been sentenced for chewing gum.

He was waiting for my reaction, and it was not long in coming—internally, at least. Several rather unempathetic responses rose to my lips. "Maybe you could have thought of that before you beat that woman half to death" was one. "If you don't wanna do the time, don't do the crime," was another.

And then I had a moment of clarity. I remembered I was in a maximum security prison. In fact, it was the closest thing to a Supermax prison that particular penal system had at the time. To be specific, I was in the segregation unit of a maximum security institution because the man in front of me was too dangerous to be kept in the regular maximum security among other inmates. He had a habit of attacking anyone—staff or inmates—he felt was annoying him, and he seemed to feel annoyed quite a bit. I remembered too that he once attacked seven police officers in an elevator, the very definition of a no-win situation.

In my moment of clarity, I realized I was in a glass room because the staff didn't trust this man in a room alone with staff, given his habit of coming over the table at them if they said the wrong thing. He was shackled, but nonetheless there was a guard outside who stayed within three feet of the door at all times. The offender had been placed within three feet of the door on the inside. That meant he was between me and the door, an arrangement I was not happy about given I was reasonably sure I could run faster than Marion Jones, depending of course on who was chasing me. But the bottom line is that security didn't want to be more than six feet away from this man when he was with a staff member, and they wanted to be able to see him at all times.

These were unusual arrangements. They are extremely labor-intensive for the staff, and prisons don't make such arrangements lightly. In fact, I can't ever remember interviewing anyone who had earned this kind of security.

And I was about to make a smart-ass comment.

The smart-ass gene in my family tree and my feminist soul argued silently for a moment with this sudden rush of clarity, and I had to choose: speak up or shut up. I have a lifetime aversion to shutting up, and normally when I err, it's on the "speak up" side of things. I thought about it for a moment.

I decided I could write him a letter if I felt strongly about this. As a character in one of my books said, "I'm either growing up or wearing down. Sometimes it's hard to tell the difference."

6

Sadists

Sadists are the sex offenders we fear most, and rightly so. The acts they commit are brutal beyond description, inhumane in the true sense of the word, and senseless to those without their particular type of hunger. The research literature describes numerous examples:

A man shot off a teenage girl's arm for the sexual thrill it gave him.[1]

A rapist of thirteen-year-old girls preferred to anally rape them on cement floors so the rapes would be more painful.[2]

A serial killer would smother his wife with a plastic bag until she passed out and then would have sex [with her]. He beat her with belts and burned her with cigarettes.[3]

A father used lit candles to cauterize the cuts he would inflict to his daughter's vagina and around her nipples.[4]

A father who knew his nine-year-old daughter was afraid of the dark tied her to a tree in the woods and allowed different cronies to come out of the woods and rape her during the night.[5]

The definition of *sexual sadism* is sexual attraction to pain, suffering, terror, or humiliation: simply put, sadists hurt people for the sexual thrill it gives them. They don't just rape people: They torture them. Sadists are not common, fortunately, even among sex offenders. Roughly 2 to 5 percent of sex offenders across studies are sadistic.[6] There is no way to discuss the dynamics of sadists, certainly no way to use their own words, without producing material that is deeply offensive. You alone know whether this material is something you should read or not.

It has the power to traumatize, and based on history and temperament, it may or may not be something you can or want to tolerate. Once during a lecture to medical students, I showed an educational film I'd made of interviews with sadists. I thought because they dissected corpses, they could tolerate the material. The students flooded the dean's office afterward in tears, and I was asked to come back and debrief them.

If this is not something you want to read, you can skip this chapter, and the rest of the book will still make sense. To be honest, you'll like the world more if you don't read it.

Sounds Outside the Normal Range

Even if we don't understand how anyone could commit a sexual assault, surely we understand at least some of the underlying drives— loneliness, sexual interest, anger—before they take a deviant bent. Having experienced sexual arousal ourselves, we can at least know what feelings child molesters are talking about, even if our sexual attraction is to adults and theirs to children. And everyone knows loneliness and perhaps can imagine what life would be like if we had somehow fastened on sex with children as an antidote.

But there are others whose motivations elude us entirely. If most of us saw a child being tortured, we would likely vomit. Compare that with this description by a sadist I will call Mr. Johnson, who repeatedly suffocated his nine-year-old stepson:

> After about two years of molesting my son, and all the pornography that I had been buying, renting, swapping, I had got my hands on some bondage discipline pornography with children involved. Some of the reading that I had done and the pictures that I had seen showed total submission. Forcing the children to do what I wanted.
>
> And I had eventually started using some of this bondage and discipline with my own son, and it had escalated to the point where I was putting a large Ziploc bag over his head and taping it

around his neck with black duct tape or black electrical tape and raping and molesting him at that point to the point that he would turn blue, pass out. At that point I would rip the bag off his head, not for fear of hurting him, but because of the excitement.

I was extremely aroused by inflicting pain. And when I see him pass out and change colors, that was very arousing and heightening to me, and I would rip the bag off his head and then I'd jump up on his chest and masturbate in his face and make him suck my penis while he was, as he started to come back awake. While he was coughing and choking, I would rape him in the mouth.

I used this same sadistic style of the plastic bag and the tape two or three times a week, and it went on for I'd say a little over a year.

Just as there are sounds many humans cannot hear but some other species can, this man has motivations, feelings, and hungers outside the normal range. If we can at least empathize with a child molester's loneliness, we cannot empathize with much of anything about a sadist: We will never know, fortunately, what it feels like to find torturing a child exciting.

Sadists may feel aroused by sexual violence, but more surprisingly, they may be sexually excited by violence alone. For example, consider a sadist who listened to a graphic story of consenting sex but had only 17 percent of an erection, compared to 61 percent of an erection to a story of rape.[7] However, when sex was removed entirely from the scenario and the description was simply of a man beating up a woman, the offender's sexual arousal went up to 79 percent. In that particular sadist's case, sex in any form actually decreased his arousal. He was most excited by pure violence.

This is not true of every sadist—some are aroused specifically by *sexual* violence. But for other sadists, it is violence toward a particular gender that is sexually stimulating, not an attack on the sex organs per se. Some of what is labeled domestic violence is sadistic abuse in disguise. Some of what is thought to be child physical abuse is sadistic abuse in disguise. Sadistic abuse is often missed because the focus is on what part of the victim's body is hurt rather than on the motivation for the assault.

Given that we don't have the same feelings as sadists, we must talk to those who do if we want to understand enough to know how to find sadists and how to stop them. Very few sadists will agree to talk. They know full well how the rest of us feel about what they do. Whereas child molesters often delude themselves into thinking that everyone, deep down, has the same interests they do, and whereas rapists feel justified in their behavior, sadists don't seem to fool themselves in the same ways. The man below, for example, fully understood how deviant his impulses were.

Finally, one day I decided I was this way. I was going to continue to be this way, and if I was going to hurt people, I was going to hurt them. I'd already made up my mind that I was going to victimize until someone killed me. Or I got locked up.

Q. You said "this way"? You mean violent? Wanting to do something violent?

A. Evil. I believed myself evil. Possessed by a demon sometimes. Anything to justify my actions.

But occasionally, sadists still agree to interviews. I'm not always sure why they do so except that some of them see interviews as an opportunity to traumatize the interviewer vicariously. It may not be as satisfying as actually torturing someone, but seeing the shock and distress others feel at their stories still feeds their hunger.

The Sadistic High

There are surprises in the interviews I have done. Although the official definition of sadism by DSM-IV—TR, the *Diagnostic and Statistical Manual of the American Psychiatric Association,* stresses *sexual* attraction to pain and suffering,[8] in fact, I have been impressed by how often sadists themselves talk about a generalized high that seems less focused on the genitals and is more like the kind of high that drugs produce.

For example, consider the following description by Mr. Carron, the offender described in Chapter 5, who abducted a woman from a convenience store. He is described in this section on sadists because he not only planned on raping his victim but also was actively considering killing her for the high he thought it would bring.

> When I stuck the pistol in my victim's back, the adrenaline rush that I got out of that—I had done drugs before, and I had drank alcohol. Nothing can compare with that rush that I got when I stuck that pistol in her back. It was like my whole world turned upside down. Everything went in slow motion for a few minutes. A lot of times I thought that I was a junkie on my own adrenaline. May not have been. It may have been other chemicals in my body. But I learned how to tap into those things by using my own fear, other people's fears, and a lot of it came with the deviant behavior. That's the only way I could tap into it. I wanted that high.

I asked if he expected it.

> The high that I got during that crime surprised me. When I stuck that pistol in her back, I almost passed out, the rush was so intense. And it scared me. Because I had already pulled a gun on this woman and stuck it in her back and for me to pass out, it scared me. I hadn't anticipated that. Not at all. I thought I would get a high but not like that.

Mr. Carron took his victim to a storage area he had prepared and tied her up with duct tape. But before he could carry through on the rest of his plan, he was tripped up by two police officers who saw a car where they didn't expect one and went to investigate. It was just a routine check and pure luck that he was apprehended. I asked Mr. Carron what would have happened had he not been caught.

> Killing my victim would have been the next high for me. The progress of my deviant behavior was highs. I went from one to another. It was an adrenaline rush for me. I wanted that rush. I had

to have it. That's what my thinking was. And the night I committed my crime, when I stuck that pistol in my victim's back, I got a rush like I had never gotten before. After that, everything had went downhill for me. I was feeling worse about it. Sometimes I questioned if I would have continued. After that, I thought the rape may not be anything. You know. But I thought, if I kill my victim, now that would be a real high.

Other sadists have also described this high. Mr. Johnson, the sadist who suffocated his son, tells me,

I'd have to say I did get a high out of violent behavior. I got—I got a high out of any controlling and dominating situation. Any, any situation that I was able to control—right?—I got a high out of. I had like an adrenaline rush. I felt powerful, in charge, where in a consensual sexual relationship, sure, orgasm was achieved, ejaculation was achieved, and then it's over. But the feeling of power and control lasts, it would last a lot longer. And it's something I knew that I could achieve at any given point in time. All I, I knew what I had to do. All I had to do was control somebody or dominate, and that high was there.

Q. Is the high from sadistic acts the same or different?

A. The high from sadistic acts is different. It's more extreme. It was more extreme. It seemed to me that committing a sadistic act and having sex involved in that sadistic act just heightened everything more: the feelings, the orgasm, the ejaculation. It seemed to heighten it even more.

This high is most commonly triggered by physical torture but not always. An offender was described in Chapter 2, one who persuaded a correctional officer to let him live with him and his family after his release from prison. This man molested the officer's nine-year-old daughter, but his motivation was not simply to molest the child. He was far more interested in setting up the family and betraying them. It was emotional torture that thrilled him. He had a long history of betraying people for the thrill it brought him, and he had no history of being physically violent.

> Getting the person to trust me first. Then I knew I could do whatever I wanted. I wanted to see the pain I could cause them, the bringing them down. It was the ultimate rush. . . .
>
> It's like a rush. I really don't know how to explain it. I've never been into drugs real strong. From just what I have seen, it's like someone addicted to heroin or cocaine. An incredible feeling. Strongest at the end when I know I'm going to let them down in some way. . . .
>
> What I felt is when you hurt somebody physically, that goes away. When you hurt somebody emotionally, that's never going to go away. That was the thrill.

The high sadists talk about is likely to explain sadistic behavior far more than any psychoanalytic theories about the abuse they may have suffered. Sadism looks and sounds like a drug addiction, albeit an internal one and one whose origins we don't understand at all. Although such a possibility has been little researched beyond interviews with sadists and thus is not proven, these men may have learned to trigger internal chemicals through violent fantasy and eventually through violent behavior.

If so, it appears the chemicals work the way many drugs do: They require stronger and stronger doses to produce the same high. The escalation seems built in. One child molester—who admitted to being aroused by pain but claimed never to have acted on it—put it this way.

> I do believe, though, if I had allowed my fantasies to become a reality as far as being violent with the children, I do sincerely believe that over time it would have become increasingly more violent and more violent and even possibly to the point of death.
>
> . . . One thing reinforces the other and brings about the next. It has to, something has to get more exciting than that, or it's just totally worthless.

This offender's entire history is of nonviolent, manipulated sex with boys. Yet I do not doubt that he was in danger of metamorphosing into a sadist. The fantasies always lead, and his fantasies had already turned sadistic.

Not every rapist or child molester turns into a sadist—most don't—but for those who do, the process often seems to be gradual, to unfold slowly over a period of years. Fantasies play a crucial role. Mr. Morgan, described in Chapter 5, talks below about how attracted he was to sexual violence. He describes too how his violent fantasies escalated over the years:

> The violence in the rape itself excites me. In my mind my fantasy is that I'm a big stud, and she's not going to be able to hold my erect penis. Therefore, she would be in a lot of pain, and the violence excites me in that aspect very much. I get a big rush off that more than I possibly, more than I do the actual assault. . . . To hear her cry or to holler that it was hurting excited me.

In prison, his fantasies have increasingly turned to children, but the emphasis on hurting has not changed.

> When I come to prison . . . I started viewing pornography more and more and more . . . fantasizing about when to hurt the individual . . . masturbating constantly to images of children—fully penetrating young children for the sole purpose of them hollering and responding that they were hurting.

Mr. Morgan used weapons as part of his offenses, and they have also been a part of his fantasies. But for him they were never the most important part. Neither was power and control. His leanings have steadily taken an increasingly sadistic path.

> The excitement of holding a weapon or a knife or forcing someone into a sexual act is exciting to me, but for me it's not the most exciting. I used the weapons primarily to force the individuals into committing the acts I wanted. I got my excitement from their

struggle, from my penetration of them more than I got from pulling the weapon on them. The weapon for me was just a mechanism to get to what excited me. Which was hurting them sexually.

But hurting them was really just the beginning of his fantasies, not the end. Over time the violence in his fantasies has continued to escalate.

It's like a step ladder. It just gets worse and worse and worse because you have to have more fuel to get the high. It's like a heroin addict. After a certain period, the dosage that he's taking has to be increased in order for him to get the same high. So it's hard for me to predict where it would go. I know they would go into the area of the victim experiencing pain from my penetration of their vagina or anus. It would probably, it would be safe to say that it would go into the sadistic, torture or sadistic swing of beating, things of this, that nature. Probably resulting in death.

The irony of this, of course, is that because so much of what happens is inside an offender's head, it makes it very difficult to profile them from their records alone. When this man is released from prison, he will be viewed by authorities as a man with a history of raping adolescent females, a man with no history of molesting young boys, certainly no history of torture. But over the years, his fantasies have changed from teenage girls to preteen boys and from rape to murder. If a seven- to nine-year-old boy is found tortured to death, this man will not even be on their list of suspects.

It is hard to describe the intensity of the fantasies that offenders develop, to appreciate how much the fantasies dominate their lives or how much they will give up to keep them. But these fantasies take on a life of their own. What starts as daydreaming eventually becomes something the offenders can't control, even when they try. Mr. Carron tells us:

My fantasies became a lot more intense as I grew older. The more I'd masturbate, the more deviant the behavior. . . . A lot of times I thought I could use self-will to stop myself. For a period of time it worked. But what it did was build up more turmoil in me. I struggled with it. And my fantasies got worse and worse. I got worse and worse. I didn't reach out for help. I didn't ask anybody for help. I didn't want it. I wanted to be doing this.

What would stop a man like this? Not much. As you can see below from Mr. Carron, neither the threat of jail nor the possibility of dying had any power to deter him. The threat of jail only made him consider killing his victim.

I see no future for myself. I had already tried to commit suicide once. I didn't want to live. But I wanted to continue to be deviant because that's the only excitement I got out of life. I seen myself, if I hadn't got caught I would have killed my victim. For me, that was my final choice. I had to kill the victim. No victim, no crime. I was uncomfortable with that while I was committing my crime. I didn't want to do that. But I kept telling myself I had to. Someone would find me out, and I wouldn't be able to continue. The night that I committed my crime, I went out of the house thinking that I'm going to do this. I'm going to do this the best I can, and I'm not going to stop until someone puts a bullet in my head.

Was the only reason he was planning on killing his victim the fear of detection? I think not. He has already admitted that he thought it would be the ultimate high. But I take him seriously that his desire to continue was intense enough that he would have killed for that reason alone. And I take seriously as well his statement that he was willing to die for the high.

Does Everybody Know What Empathy Is?

It is not just the presence of a high in these cases that is surprising. It is also the absence of empathy, of any concern for these victims. How could you or I treat another human being like this? Mr. Johnson, the man who suffocated his son, responds:

At the time I didn't have any feelings for anybody other than myself. I wanted me to feel good. And it didn't make a difference who hurt in the process as long as I felt good. . . .

At that point in my life, I don't think I had empathy for anybody. . . . I'm not even sure I knew what empathy was at that point. I didn't care about other people's feelings. I didn't care for other people. Period. I really don't believe that I, that I really understood what empathy was at that time.

Callousness is routine in sadists. Note, for example, that the sadist below had no real sexual interest in children, but he also had no compunction about the idea of attacking one for practice.

The picture in my mind was one of torturing a victim with everything from matches to cigarette butts to a propane torch, electrical stimulation, needles, and so forth. . . . The first few victims were female because I had an impulse to rape and hurt. The last three were female for rape reasons, but with more emphasis on hurting and humiliation. . . . And, on a few occasions, there have been concepts of taking a "dry run" or a practice run using a small child as victim, male or female.[9]

When you ask sadists about callousness toward people, they often shrug and tell you that they treated people as objects. Witness Mr. Carron's response below:

I told myself that she was an object a lot. I told myself everybody was an object. I had stayed so out of touch with reality and stayed away from so many others for so long, masturbating and fantasizing, I had built up a world within my mind that no one was real but me. And I could do whatever I wanted to. And the only enjoyment that I had out of life was the adrenaline rush I got when I done or participated in deviant behavior.

But there is more to this than these men say. If they had truly felt these people were objects, they would not have attacked them. Sadists don't attack trees or cars. The point is that they are acutely aware of how people feel. Unlike the rageful rapist who vents anger with no real knowledge or caring about how the victim feels, sadists do not explode in a frenzied, violent attack; instead, they slowly torture. They torture, listening carefully to how the person feels and adjusting the torture to increase the suffering.

The point of sadism is not indifference to pain. It is the deliberate infliction of pain and terror. Sadists will often blindfold their victims, even when they are planning to kill them, in order to induce terror.[10] Often sadists will tell their victims in advance what will happen to them in order to increase the terror. One serial killer would say to his victims:

> First, I'm going to torture you in the most horrible and painful manner I can think of. Then I'm going to abuse you sexually in the most degrading way I possibly can think of. Then I'll kill you in the slowest and most painful way I can conceive. . . . Do you have any questions?[11]

What fuels sadists then is not a belief that people are objects but rather a kind of reverse empathy. Rather than being indifferent to how others feel, they are exquisitely attuned to it. But suffering in others does not produce the same feeling state in them. Instead, it produces its opposite. Other people's helplessness makes them feel powerful. Other people's vulnerability makes them feel invincible. Other people's dying makes them feel alive. Other people's submission makes them feel dominant. When you or I see someone in pain, we empathize, which is to say, we feel some of that pain ourselves. Sadists feel satisfied, high, happy instead.

Consider, for example, the offender who attacked an eleven-year-old girl, raped her, bound her hands and feet, tied a rope around her neck, and dragged her across an open field until she passed out. Thinking she was dead, he left her. Later, he was caught and admitted to the offense. When asked how he felt at the time, he said, "Like Superman: strong, invincible and horny, too!"[12]

A lack of empathy is not peculiar to sadists: Violent rapists, many child molesters, and all psychopaths share it. But what is peculiar to sadists is this feeding off of the pain. Psychopaths, violent rapists, and many child molesters just ignore the pain of others. It is irrelevant, and they do not mind causing it in the service of their own enjoyment. Rapists certainly intend to inflict pain. But even rapists do not inflict pain slowly, deliberately, devouring the victim's response like someone having a gourmet meal.

Perhaps vampires exist after all, except that they do not literally drink the victim's blood. Indeed, Bram Stoker, the author of the original story, took the name Dracula from accounts of a fifteenth-century sadist named Vlad the Impaler, also known as Dracula. There is no evidence that Vlad the Impaler actually drank the blood of his victims, although he shed plenty of it, impaling as many as 20,000 people at a time. But Stoker was figuratively correct, if not literally. Vampires seem merely a metaphor for this most dangerous and harmful of human beings, the kind who emotionally drinks in the suffering of others.

Rationales, Excuses, and Further Proof of Human Ingenuity

Like most sex offenders, sadists often justify their behavior. But what possible excuses could anybody use to justify torture? When I ask audiences this, they grow thoughtful. It is a daunting task for normal people to find excuses for the inexcusable.

The sadists I have talked with, however, have no such difficulty. Some convince themselves that their victims aren't really suffering that much, and in any case, their victims actually want this to happen.

If a child was screaming, I would tell myself—you know—the child's not really hurting because I know that in reality I was hurting the child. But the only way I could continue the act was to tell myself I wasn't hurting the child. I really wasn't hurting him. I found the more I told myself that, the more I believed it. And then I found that if the child tried to pull away, or screamed, hollered, cried, then all my lying to myself would enhance it, and made it more arousing to me. And the pain, the aspect of inflicting pain, was extremely arousing.

It was something that had taken time to build up. It didn't just happen. It took time to build that up. And after a while, I could actually take it and turn it around. Because the child was screaming that he wanted more—actually because they liked it. The child was screaming because he wanted me to continue. And it's all turning it around and saying that the tears, really they aren't real for hurt. The screaming, it isn't really because of the pain. It's that the person actually wants this to happen. And that's how I was turning it around. And I told myself this so many times that I believed it.

Sitting in this interview, I found myself hard pressed to understand what this man was talking about and, frankly, hard pressed to listen. How could he tell himself it was and wasn't hurting the child at the same time? But the mind is ingenious, and its ingenuity can be used to support evil as easily as good. Initially, he separated the two perceptions. Only later was he able to do the more complicated juggling act of keeping both in mind at the same time.

When I first found that I was really aroused by inflicting pain, I didn't have that line of thinking right then, OK? I knew that I was hurting them. It took me some time, and I worked it through at a later time. I'd work it over a half hour, forty-five minutes, an hour and a half, that this child was asking for it, that he wanted more. And the more I looked at it this way, there came a point in my life, after six or seven months of doing it, that I didn't even have to change the thought process any more. The immediate thought process was scream, pain, excitement: They wanted it. There was no change after that.

Other sadists do not bother with such elaborate excuses. A more common justification is simply to say the child is disgusting, evil, sick, perverted; he deserves the treatment he receives.

I devalued all of them. All children—mostly others and my stepchild. I said, I told myself that my stepchild, because he wasn't mine, being as he wasn't my biological son, that he was less than human anyway. Other people's children that I had raped and molested, they weren't mine. They weren't my biological children, so it didn't make any difference to me. I viewed children as a piece of meat. To me children were a toy. Do what I wanted with and then throw it away.

Even today, after working with the tape of that interview for several years, I cannot hear him call children "a piece of meat" without anger. But at least the wave of homicidal rage that used to sweep over me each and every time has finally lessened. The certainty in my soul that this man has forfeited his right to walk on this planet has not.

Despite his statement, do not be tempted to think he is telling the truth when he implies he treated his biological children any better. They were younger and were just moving into the age range he preferred as victims. He admitted to me that he was getting ready to molest them and that he had gotten them to the point where it would be easy. His preparation, he stated matter-of-factly, consisted of beating and threatening to kill them to the point that they were too afraid to resist anything he told them to do. No doubt he would simply have a different excuse for molesting them.

This type of excuse, that the victim is somehow evil or defective or "less than human," is simply projection. The father of one of my clients told her she was too egocentric to ever have children. Another sadistic father told his daughter/victim that she didn't feel things but only pretended to. Someone was, indeed, too egocentric to have children in that house, and someone didn't feel things. Someone was also less than human, but in no case was it the child.

This process of projection is the same one that nonsadistic child molesters use, projection of the offender's inner world onto the victim. The difference is in what lies within. For the nonsadistic child molester, it is sexual arousal to children that comprises his inner world, and that is what he projects outward onto the child. He believes the child desires sex with him. The sadist projects a sense of evil, of extreme perversion. The evil that lies within he throws away from him, onto the child. These are truly "people of the lie."

But of course, all of these projections rely on the perpetrator having some prior contact with the victim. But what do those who prey on strangers tell themselves?

Some denigrate whole classes of people, such as women or children. Many rapists believe that women are "bitches" who deserve anything bad that happens to them. Those who attack children employ similarly distorted cognitions in regard to children. "I think young girls and boys are meant to be sex slaves or sex playthings for adults" was the statement of one sadistic offender, writing to someone he thought was another pedophile—in reality, a federal marshal running a sting operation.

Ted Bundy only admitted he was a murderer shortly before he was executed, but even before then, he spoke about the murders in the third person to two journalists who interviewed him.[13] While maintaining his innocence, he allowed that, nevertheless, he could put himself in the mind of the killer and tell them what such a man *might* think and feel. Under this rather thin cover, he talked about his way of operating and his justifications. He described "the killer" as being "amazed and chagrined" at the public outcry that followed the disappearance of a victim. Why would anyone pay so much attention? He said the killer told himself, "What's one less? . . . What's one less person on the face of the planet? What difference will it make a hundred years from now?"[14] After all, "people disappear every day! It happens all the time. . . . I mean, there are *so* many people. This person will never be missed. It shouldn't be a problem."[15]

In that statement Bundy revealed that he never grasped the concept of attachment, that one person could care about another, could miss them, might even grieve. But if he valued no one else's life, he seems to have been attached to his own. Before he died, he decided capital punishment was unfair. It was wrong, he said, for the state to kill people. Clearly, his sense of irony was as deficient as his conscience.

Some part of my vindictive little soul wanted to be there. Not for the execution—I have no taste for killing. Only to say to him beforehand,

"But Ted, people disappear every day! It happens all the time. After all, there are *so* many people. I don't think you will ever be missed. It shouldn't be a problem."

Would I have said it? I don't know. It is at odds with the notion I cling to that how you treat people should come from who you are, not who they are. But I would have been sorely tempted.

Who Are They?

If you think that the sadists and the Ted Bundys of the world must somehow look different and can be spotted on the street, think again. Despite an extraordinary level of deviancy and callousness, they are often well ensconced in communities. Many sadists are what former FBI agent Roy Hazelwood has termed "three piece suit offenders. . . . One was a churchman, another worked as a high-level executive for a Midwest chain. One guy was an ex-cop." Some of the worst were "pillars of the community."[16]

If you were attacked by a sadist, you'd not likely identify him by going through mug shots. In one study, 65 percent had no prior record.[17] Those sadists who were termed "more severe" (defined as killing three or more people) were considerably better adjusted and more successful than those termed "less severe" (defined as killing only one person), according to one study.[18] For example, 43 percent of the more severe sadists were married at the time of the offense, as opposed to 7 percent of the less severe ones; 33 percent had military experience as opposed to none of the less severe; 43 percent had education beyond high school as compared to none; and a full one-third had a reputation as a solid citizen, as opposed to none of the less severe.

It is not likely that these results are because of the fact that being middle class makes someone a more severe sadist. It is more likely that being a pillar of the community means they didn't get caught right away. After all, when there is a particularly gruesome murder in a small town, who looks at a local school teacher, a well-known psychologist, or a doctor with no criminal record as a possible suspect?

However, even middle class sadists with no criminal records often leave a trail of sorts. First of all, as many as 65 percent of sadists keep trophies, such mementos of their victims as a lock of hair or a driver's license, and 45 percent video- or audiorecord their offenses.[19] It is always useful to get a search warrant when investigating a sadist.

Wives and Girlfriends

If the outside world doesn't know who sadists are, their partners often do. Sadists will try out the behaviors they use on victims outside the home initially on wives and girlfriends in the home. However, even those who kill people outside the home usually do not kill their partners. There is simply too much risk of detection, and sadists tend to be excellent planners.

I mentioned previously a man who had raped and killed a neighbor child who came to his door on Halloween. In going through the records, I found that years before he had picked up a former girlfriend in a bar one night. He saw her sitting alone and crying because she had broken up with her current beau (a different man). He offered her a ride home, but instead of taking her home, he drove her to an isolated area and raped her anally with such violence that she vomited throughout the attack. He continued nonetheless, his sexual interest undeterred—and perhaps enhanced—by her distress.

This is consistent with his behavior the night the child was killed. He had sent his wife to a Halloween party alone, claiming he didn't feel well. While she was gone, the child came trick-or-treating. He killed the little girl, put her body in a garbage bag, and hid it temporarily in the basement. When his wife returned, he was so sexually aroused that he demanded sex, a fact that stood in stark contrast to his later claim that he killed the child accidentally. In reality, it is highly unlikely that anyone who accidentally killed a child would find the event sexually exciting.

If you're wondering why anyone would marry a sadist, it's because sadists do not announce themselves when courting. In fact, according to research by Hazelwood, it appears that sadists present initially as exactly the opposite of what they are.[20] In a study of partners of serial killers, Hazelwood found that they frequently begin relationships by showering prospective partners with attention and affection. It seems a caricature of normal courting, as though the offender were trying to present as some kind of idealized figure picked up from a romance novel.

He will give small gifts, be unusually sensitive and attentive, profess his undying love early on—heady stuff for the woman who believes she has found the romance she has been waiting for, the one the books say is just around the corner, the one in the fairy tales.

At some point, the couple becomes sexually intimate, and things go well for a time. But eventually the offender will discover some sort of sex his partner does not enjoy. Rather than drop it, he will insist on it. It doesn't matter what form of sex it is. If the woman enjoys anal sex but does not like oral sex, it will be oral sex. If she enjoys oral sex but not anal, it will be anal. The point is simply to find something that the wife or girlfriend does not like.

As the relationship develops, the demands for the unwanted sex acts escalate while the types of sex the woman enjoys drop out. At this point the offender will begin isolating his partner, cutting her off from friends and family and demanding she spend all of her time with him. Sooner or later, after social isolation comes torture and virtual captivity. By the time the torture begins, the woman is demoralized, isolated, and worn down. She also may have been beaten repeatedly, often to the point of unconsciousness.

The sexual torture is elaborate and usually ritualistic, by which I mean that the same things are done in a precise sequence every time. The ritual is "scripted," planned out in detail, and the husband may spend hours explaining the exact sequence to his wife and what she will be required to do. For instance, one woman was forced to come in the house barefoot and brush her hair in front of a mirror while the husband crept up behind her and grabbed her around the neck. She was told her eyes had to widen just so in surprise. He would then drag her off to the bedroom where he had rings fastened in the wall to immobilize her. He would torture her in a particular sequence and then strangle her into unconsciousness. This was her sex life for eight years.

Each particular sadist will have a different script, with elements of force, torture, and control as the only constants. There is no spontaneity in this sequence. All aspects of sadistic offenses tend to be planned, both inside and outside the home.

Michael DeBardeleben, a counterfeiter and sadist, was one of those who kept voluminous notes on his exploits. Among the notes was found his recipe for a relationship:

A [man] must be aware of all this:
   —Get his satisfaction early
   —Isolate her contacts with others
   —Don't let her make *any* decisions
   —Don't let her acquire any skills (working, driving, social skills, etc.)
   —Don't let her have any power (bank accounts, ownership, inside information—material for blackmail)
   —*Never* trust her completely
   —Don't "enlighten" her with knowledge (especially of psychology)
   —Always remember that the relationship is *temporary* + likewise prepare to "cut her loose" before she does it to you
   —Set the "price" higher than needed at first; whip, infidelity, extreme humiliation—then gradually reduce to keep at an adequate level
   —Actively seek a "new" partner when she begins to show signs of rebellion
   —Make her more dependent: drugs? Live in country. No phone (or hidden—for my use only) no drivers license, no books (except fantasy) no fancy clothes, no doctors
   —*Never* show weakness, guilt or insecurity.[21]

Once I was lecturing on sadism, and a woman lingered after the lecture to speak with me. After all the other questions had been answered and the other participants gone, she told me this tale from many years ago. She was eighteen years old at the time, living in Rochester, New

York. One day she was shopping with a friend when a security guard approached her in the store. He was polite, well mannered, and somewhat diffident, and he struck up a conversation with her and her friend. She liked him, and at the end of the conversation he asked her for her phone number; she gave it.

He called soon thereafter and asked her out. He was courteous in the extreme, and they began dating. Very quickly, he appeared to fall head-over-heels for her. She worked as a teller in the bank, and he began showing up at the bank to put a fresh loaf of bread or flowers through the drive-up window. All the other tellers thought he was someone out of *An Officer and a Gentleman.* They told her she should marry him.

She was not so sure. He seemed to be moving much too fast, more smothering her than going out with her. Within a few weeks, he wanted to move in, but she refused. She needed more time.

Still, she liked him, enjoyed going out with him, and had no suspicions that he had any sort of dark side. He did talk about his "evil twin," a twin brother who supposedly was always in trouble, but she believed the "twin" was real.

Then one day the buzzer to her apartment rang. She opened the door to find a large sculpture sitting there. The sculpture was made of wire and featured twisted, clawing hands and a face screaming horribly. It shocked her, as no doubt it was meant to, and she grabbed it and dragged it inside, embarrassed that the neighbors might see it. Interestingly, she knew immediately who left it there.

She called her "admirer," and when she got through, he admitted it was he who had left the sculpture but gave a lame excuse. He needed a place to store the sculpture and thought she might be willing. He had no explanation for why he hadn't talked to her about it first.

This was too much for her. Already feeling that he was pushing her for too much, too soon, she broke up with him. A year went by in which there was no contact. She renewed her relationship with another man, but they, too, broke up. On the night of the break-up, she drove home, upset and crying, and she didn't notice a car that pulled up next to her at the stoplight. The driver of that car rolled down his window and spoke to her. It was her former friend. He seemed concerned and asked her what was wrong.

She was part way through telling him when the light changed. She remembered him as someone who had never hurt her, and indeed, he never had. She had no hesitation in inviting him back to her apartment for coffee.

When they got there, he brutally raped her. Afterward, she lay sobbing on the couch while he sat on the sofa next to her staring at the floor. She reported his expression was completely blank, a look she had never seen before. Without a word, he got up and walked out.

She never saw him again. At least not in person. But ten years later, she turned on the news and discovered that he had become the Hillside Strangler.

I have no way of knowing if this story is true. I do not know her name, and I never saw her again. But the story does have the ring of truth. The courting process she described is one in which sadists engage. Also, Kenneth Bianco, the Hillside Strangler, tried, when he was caught, to throw the blame onto an "evil twin" or alter ego named Steven Walker, claiming he had multiple personality disorder. It is also true that he lived in Rochester, New York, until he was twenty-six years old, and true too that while there, he worked as a security guard.

You would think that knowing all this, I would not underestimate offenders, but at times I have. Once I was shooting an educational film in a prison when there was a "miscount." Prisons count all their inmates several times a day, and if the right number doesn't come up, all programming shuts down while they count again. Almost always the problem is literally a miscount, but every miscount has to be treated as a possible escape until proven otherwise. This miscount came when I was in the middle of a confrontation with an inmate about his denial. I was left unsettled by the unfinished interview, and I came back that night, with permission from prison authorities, to complete the interview.

I did not have the film crew with me this time. They were setting up at another site for the next day's filming, and I was alone. I expected the staff member who met me at the gate to accompany me, but she went home. I was not on monitor. Instead, I was alone with this inmate, several locked steel doors from the nearest guard. This was not one of my smarter moments.

In my defense, I was aware the man I was there to see was coming up for parole. I had read his records and did not think for a second that he was an impulsive offender. I thought he planned everything he ever did, and I did not think he would want to do anything that would hurt his chance of parole. It turns out I was underestimating how much I can annoy people.

The man was good-looking, well educated, and well spoken. He had been a respected veterinarian in his community. He did not look like most people's idea of a criminal, and you would most certainly not be afraid of him on sight.

He had three known offenses to date. The first occurred when he picked up his thirteen-year-old daughter, ostensibly to take her to the hospital to visit her mother, who was having a hysterectomy that day. Instead, he suddenly grabbed a syringe lying on the dashboard and injected her in the thigh with Demerol, then disappeared with her until the next day. No one knows what happened.

He admits he did this but claims it wasn't an offense and that nothing happened in the missing twenty-four hours. He only wanted to stop the surgery, he said, which he had opposed. He claimed not to understand why he was charged and convicted of assault for such a little thing. His explanation doesn't make any sense, particularly in the light of his other offenses, but we move on.

His second offense was to run into a YMCA women's dressing room, where he found a thirteen-year-old girl alone. He denies following her or stalking her, but it strains coincidence to think he could simply walk into a YMCA dressing room randomly and find a victim of his preferred age and sex alone.

He grabbed this girl and injected her with an animal sedative, but she broke free of him and ran to the lobby before she collapsed. He was convicted, but the case was overturned on a technicality: The line-up of photos wasn't properly presented. He would not discuss this offense because he denies he did it. But to believe him, we have to believe there was more than one man running around injecting thirteen-year-old girls with sedatives in his rural community.

His third offense involved breaking into an apartment where a thirteen-year-old girl was alone. He admitted going into the apartment, but again, he denied planning this offense or stalking the girl and claimed that the fact that a thirteen-year-old girl was home alone when he went into the apartment was merely an accident. In fact, he denied that he even broke in. The door was open, he says, and he only walked in to ask for directions—something anyone would do.

The stabbing, he claimed, was another accident. He admitted he forced the girl to strip at the point of a knife. Afterward, he said, she made a dash for the door and impaled herself on his knife. I looked down at the police report in my hands. The girl was stabbed in the back. To believe him I must believe she tried to escape by running backward, nude, toward her attacker.

He was still angry that he was incarcerated for that offense. "An irrational two minutes of my life," he says. "Why should I spend all these years in prison for simply an irrational two minutes of my life?" He had refused treatment in prison. He didn't need treatment. It was simply an irrational two minutes, nothing to do with him.

Calmly I pointed out that if he didn't know why he did this the last time, he has no way to prevent it from happening the next time. In that case, I said, he should stay in prison forever, or if that wasn't possible, then as long as the law will allow, a statement that seemed to annoy him immensely. But he only became truly angry when in the course of this comment I used the word "sex offender." He stopped me immediately.

"Sex offender?" he said. "What makes you think I'm a sex offender?"

I was puzzled that he could even question this. "When you force someone to strip at the point of a knife," I said slowly, "that makes you a sex offender."

"But how do you know I was thinking about raping her?" he asked. "How do you know I wasn't thinking about cutting her head off."

That silenced me. "Were you?" I said quietly.

"More that," he replied, "than the other."

I paused, thinking about the fact that two twelve-year-old girls were missing in his area, and the man in front of me was a suspect. I had a sick feeling suddenly that when these two children are eventually found, they may be decapitated.

Suddenly I was overwhelmed by the futility of trying to learn anything about this man from words. The words fluttered about the room like butterflies he put out only to distract me. For just a moment in my mind's eye, I saw a bubble over his head, like a cartoon, but instead of words there was gibberish in the bubble, a fair summation of this interview thus far.

Then I had a bizarre fantasy impulse. I wanted the room to fill up with gas, as it did sometimes in old *Star Trek* episodes, gas that would freeze him in mid-sentence but not me. I wanted this to happen so that I could reach over and touch the skin on his forehead. It was some kind of primal instinct, as though I could learn through touch what I could not learn through words. How could anyone even contemplate cutting off a child's head? Was this man real? Was that skin real? Perhaps it was plastic. So alien was this man from me, I went back to some primitive need to touch.

The moment passed. I shook it off and persisted in confronting him. I told him one more time that he should be locked up forever if he couldn't take responsibility for his behavior and go into treatment to control it. Suddenly, anger seemed to seize him. He stood up abruptly and rocked back and forth on his feet. I looked up into his rage-filled face and realized he was making a decision, whether to go forward toward me or away. He could not stay where he was.

There was a second when my heart stopped, and I waited, knowing that I had lost control of this situation. Then he headed toward the door. He hit the button next to it, barked something to the guard, and I heard footsteps coming to take him back to his cell. Soon I was alone with my own stupidity.

Over and over again we underestimate these people. Over and over we expect rationality, expect motives we can understand, expect that there is some kind of agreement between us on the rules of conduct. Over and over we expect that we can ride down a country road in midday without being run off the road and raped by a sex offender, expect that we can speak sharply to a man harassing us in a McDonald's parking lot without getting attacked and raped, expect that we can be the last to close up a nature center without getting abducted and tortured—yet I have had clients who were victimized in each of those situations. Over and over we expect that we can interview a man in prison without getting hurt, a man who has everything to lose and nothing to gain by attacking anyone. Over and over, we are wrong.

7

Psychopaths: Fooling People for the Thrill of It

While sex offenders—even violent predators—have a fear of getting caught and use deception pragmatically as a way of maintaining their freedom, psychopaths—offenders without a conscience—fool people for the thrill of it. Deception is not just a byproduct of deviant activities for the psychopath; often it is the main event.

Psychopaths are predators but not necessarily sexual predators. They do whatever interests them, whether it is sexual molestation, mugging, or robbing banks. Research by Dr. Robert Hare indicates that between 15 and 25 percent of the inmates in U.S. prisons are psychopaths.[1] Obviously, what interests the ones who end up in prison is illegal, but it is not clear that all psychopaths have such a proclivity for illegal activity. There are those who are considerably more successful and who manage to stay on the right side of the law (or to avoid detection).

A study, for instance, looked at psychopaths in business.[2] In the course of working with six different companies, a business consultant named Paul Babiak discovered each had a problematic employee at the heart of their difficulties. In each case, the person scored high on psychopathy. The damage these individuals did to the company and to other employees was considerable. Their modus operandi was to gather information, to manipulate, to spread vicious rumors about other employees, and to sow dissension. The one thing they did not do was any sort of productive work.

Astonishingly, none were fired, despite the fact that in some cases they were losing massive amounts of money for the corporation, and in all cases, they were trailing a wake of complaints from other employees.

Quite the contrary, all of the psychopaths thrived. They excelled at fooling upper-level management into believing that none of the failures or complaints was due to their behavior; someone else always took the blame.

They were particularly good at not just cultivating upper-level management but also at cultivating some mid- and lower-level people who were in positions to give them access to information. Eventually, however, they betrayed many of these lower-level employees, then abandoned them abruptly, leaving their former "friends" feeling devalued and depressed. They continued to cultivate their bosses, however, until they took over their jobs and replaced them. In all of their dealings, they manifested the same lack of a conscience and lack of concern for others as did their counterparts serving hard time.

However, this kind of psychopath is not typically violent. Given that this book is concerned with violence and sexual assault, I will confine my comments to the type of psychopath who often does end up in jail. Still, it is important to remember that not having a criminal record does not guarantee that someone is not a psychopath. Many are not caught, and some lie, cheat, and deceive without getting on the wrong side of the law.

The type who does commit crimes, however, is the type of psychopath who has been most researched. Such psychopaths tend to be equal opportunity offenders, meaning that they often commit a variety of crimes. Even those who are sex offenders rarely limit themselves to sexual crimes. For example, an offender I evaluated had eleven sexual convictions, an astonishing number. However, he also had a total of twenty-five overall convictions, the remainder being for credit card fraud, car theft, and a variety of other crimes.

Psychopaths routinely start their criminal careers at a younger age than other offenders, on average beginning before the age of twelve.[3] They commit more crimes at every age than other inmates, and if they specialize in anything, it is in violent crime per se.[4] As they age, they reduce the number of nonviolent crimes they commit, but they do not decrease the number of violent crimes, the opposite pattern from other violent offenders.[5]

What is particularly sobering, however, is just how many crimes psychopaths commit and how little incarceration affects them. They are three times more likely to commit a general offense within the first year of release than other offenders and four times more likely to commit a violent offense.[6] They are truly a formidable group of criminals. They start young, commit high numbers of violent crimes with little remorse, and don't seem bothered by being caught and imprisoned.

Thugs and Charmers: The Guilty and the Guiltless

If violence were all, psychopaths would simply be thugs. But what distinguishes psychopaths from other offenders is not just their level of violence and their propensity for crime; it is that they have personality traits that allow them to manipulate people pretty much with impunity. Key characteristics of psychopathy are glibness, superficial charm, and an extraordinary ability to con and to manipulate.

But it is somehow more than that. Really good psychopaths are genuinely likable. A friend of mine recently was describing a psychopath she had known in childhood. He was the father of her best friend, and as an insurance salesman he embezzled quite a lot of money out of the people in their small town. Eventually he absconded with the money, abandoning her friend and her friend's mother. The friend's house—which he had borrowed against extensively—was repossessed by the bank. The mother became severely depressed, and the townspeople stepped in to help move the family because the mother simply wasn't coping. Her friend and her friend's mother became destitute. Eventually friends bought tickets for the family and put them on a train to meet relatives. The entire frightening, embarrassing ordeal devastated her friend's childhood and destroyed the mental health of the mother.

But after telling this dreadful tale, my friend got a dreamy look in her eyes and said, "But you know, if Jack walked through the door today, I'd be glad to see him. He was just that kind of person." She went on to talk about funny comments he had made when she was at his house as a child. She still remembered them verbatim.

Likewise, Babiak confirmed that the coworkers of the psychopaths in business who were dumped and abandoned by the psychopaths were not only angry and betrayed, they were depressed partly because they missed the psychopath and the excitement he or she had brought into their lives.[7]

Even Professor Daniel Lykken, an expert on antisocial personalities, speaks amiably of a psychopath named Duane who cheated him out of $1000, despite the fact that Lykken knew he was a psychopath from the start with a track record of criminal behavior and of lying and manipulating. Lykken's only comment was, "You would not think me quite such a fool if you had been there yourself and heard Duane's casual, low-keyed pitch, full of circumstantial detail."[8] Lykken even allowed Duane to pilot him in a small plane, despite remembering on the way to the airport that Duane was reckless, had no fear, and liked close calls.

One likely reason psychopaths can thrive in business and elsewhere is that their lying and manipulation is just so difficult to detect. Normal people feel some degree of guilt and nervousness when lying, and if they're not careful, they will show signs of that guilt in their facial expressions or body language. We assume the presence of guilt in others and routinely expect that those lying to us will be made uncomfortable by the lying. In fact, what most people look for as a sign of lying is simply nervousness, anxiety, or discomfort.

But the psychopathic mindset is different. Imagine what life would be like if every human interaction were a football play. There is no "we" between adversaries on the football field. They are competing, and the outcome is win, lose, or draw. If one wins five yards, he doesn't have to feel guilty. After all, the other guy is trying to do the same thing. Did Joe Montana or Kurt Warner ever feel bad about winning a Super Bowl? Isn't pride a more understandable feeling? And that's what psychopaths feel when they dupe you and me.

Psychopaths are misread over and over because the average person expects those who betray us to have the decency to feel bad about it. It is a sad and dangerous expectation. Instead of feeling remorse over deceiving others, psychopaths feel what is termed "duping delight," a kind of joy and almost childlike delight in duping other people. The average person misreads the joy of predation as the guilelessness of innocence. After all, there is no gaze aversion, no nervous mannerisms. Seems as though the guy is pretty straight. Why, he looked me right in the eye.

Sure he did. And the clear conscience and the lack of personal distress were genuine. In fact, look closely and you will see the same joy the professional football player has when he spikes the ball in the end zone or the exuberance a boxer has when he raises both hands over a senseless opponent. It is the joy of winning, nothing more, nothing less. The difference is that anyone entering the ring or walking onto the field knows a game is going on and what the rules are. In life, psychopaths are playing a different game with a different rule book from the rest of us.

It is important to understand fully that such offenders do not have a conscience as you and I know it. Acts that would bother others—and even haunt nonpsychopathic child molesters or rapists—give no pause, cause no regret. For instance, consider the words of the psychopath below:

Yea, it was power and control. I was grooming her from the age of . . . it started about the age of one. When . . . I was the punisher. I was the one who decided punishment over the children. I was the one who spanked the children. I was the one who punished the children. And if I seen the children doing anything wrong, even bickering, arguing among themselves, I would whip them and tell them—you know, just kids playing, I would tell myself well, she's not going to be like that. She's going to be the perfect mate. And I told myself that. And I didn't molest her then.

Q. The perfect mate.

A. The perfect mate. I was grooming her to fit me. To fit me.

Q. At what age?

A. I started at about a year. I started grooming her, whipping her, and telling her this. To do this, not to do that. Then I molested her at eighteen months old. And I thought to myself. This is going to be easy. This is going to be easy. I'm going to have my own child, my own stepdaughter, which is really not blood related to me, and I'm telling myself these things. It's not blood related to me. When she grows up to be fourteen, fifteen years old, I will have the perfect sexual mate. For sexual purposes. Anything else didn't matter. It was sex. That was it. I didn't care about, really honestly, I didn't love the child. I wanted the child for my own purposes.

Q. How would you justify it in your head?

A. How did I justify it in my head? She's going to do what I want her to do, and that's it. . . . I told her that Daddy loves her. Daddy's going to take care of her, and Daddy's going to give her anything she wants as long as she does what Daddy tells her.

The film I made of this man upsets even professional audiences. There is something about his degree of callousness toward a toddler that will suck the air out of a room. It is especially hard to watch his face: the sly smile, the sparkle in the eyes. "See how clever I am," he seems to be saying. "Ain't I something!" He is indeed, but he and I would probably disagree on what.

An Old Problem

We do not want to believe such callousness exists, but it does and always has. A sign of a robust syndrome is when it is found in vastly different time periods and cultures. Schizophrenia, major depression, and psychopathy—all can be recognized across hundreds, even thousands of years.

In fact, in looking for a case study that would illustrate all the classic features of psychopathy, I found I could do no better than a man who lived 2,400 years ago, 400 years B.C.E. He might well be the poster child for psychopathy, given how well he fits the syndrome. His name was Alcibiades, and he was a legendary general in the Golden Age of Athens. His life was described in detail by Plutarch in the first century C.E., and he was mentioned by Dr. Hervey Cleckley in his early writings on psychopaths.[9]

He was a man born to every advantage. He came from one of Athen's noblest families, and when his wealthy and honored father died, the legendary statesman Pericles became his guardian. But from the start there were signs of recklessness, of a stubborn egocentricity not found among his peers, as evidenced below:

> As he played at dice in the street, being then but a child, a loaded cart came that way, when it was his turn to throw; at first he called to the driver to stop, because he was to throw in the way over which the cart was to pass; but the man giving him no attention and driving on, when the rest of the boys divided and gave way, Alcibiades threw himself on his face before the cart and, stretching himself out, bade the carter pass on now if he would; which so startled the man, that he put back his horses, while all that saw it were terrified, and, crying out, ran out to assist Alcibiades.[10]

Carts did not stop for small boys in Athens during this time period. The boy bold enough to throw himself before the cart grew up to be a man who would betray three countries, and in so doing, all his friends, relatives, and fellow Athenians—despite the fact he was loved by his family and friends and honored in every place he went.

What seems odd, in retrospect, is how long Alcibiades got away with bad behavior and how loved he was in spite of it—odd except that this contradiction is pervasive throughout psychopathic sagas. Long before he betrayed Athens, he had a track record of abusive and violent behavior, which everyone around him ignored. His record for assault was so bad that his brother-in-law, fearful that Alcibiades would murder him for his money, announced in the Athenian Senate that if he should die without children, all his lands and money would go to the state.

He was surely right about Alcibiades's callousness. It was Alcibiades who persuaded the Athenians to attack the isle of Melos and—upon the surrender of its inhabitants—to kill all the men of an age to bear arms, an outrage even in those brutal times that the Athenians came to regret sorely.

His arrogance was as well known as his propensity for violence. He wore a long purple cloak that trailed in the dust, and he sent seven chariots to the Olympic games, more than any king or country had ever sent. Instead of the usual Athenian insignia on his shield, he drew a cupid holding a thunderbolt. To older Athenians, this was comparable to a contemporary soldier removing the U.S. insignia from his or her uniform and painting on a Day-Glo nude instead.

Once he refused a dinner invitation at the house of Anytus but showed up drunk anyway. Seeing the guests dining with gold and silver cups, he commanded his servants to grab half the cups—literally taking them out of the hands of the guests. His servants took the booty home while Alcibiades disdained to even enter the room. When the astonished guests—strangers to the area—protested, Anytus replied that Alcibiades "had shown great consideration and tenderness in taking only a part when he might have taken all."[11]

It was astonishing how much he got away with. The historian Durant wrote that he "violated a hundred laws and injured a hundred men, but no one dared bring him before a court."[12] The reason seems to be more his capacity to charm than fear of his violence. Plutarch notes that the Athenians tended to "patiently endure his excesses . . . to give the softest names to his faults, attributing them to youth and good nature."[13]

Part of this inexplicable blindness had to do with Alcibiades's looks, what Plutarch termed his "brilliant and extraordinary beauty,"[14] which apparently only improved as he got older. Part of it was his gift of persuasion. It seems Alcibiades had the "highest capacity for inventing, for discerning what was the right thing to be said for any purpose."[15] But mostly it was simply his charm. Plutarch tells us that, "even those who feared and envied him could not but take delight, and have a sort of kindness for him, when they saw him and were in his company."[16]

There was one, however, who had a better eye. Timon, a respected Athenian statesman, is alleged to have said to Alcibiades, "Go on boldly, my son, and increase in credit with the people, for thou wilt one day bring them calamities enough."[17]

Timon was right, of course. Although Alcibiades became a brilliant and successful general, he never stopped being Alcibiades, and eventually his behavior caught up with him. The trouble began when he was accused of defacing all the statues of Mercury while on a drunken spree with friends. This, at last, was something totally unacceptable to the

Athenians. They were launching a military expedition to Syracuse the next day, and they feared the gods even more than they loved Alcibiades.

Faced with a trial, Alcibiades defected to Sparta, then the archenemy of Athens. There he used his knowledge of the Athenian military to advise their bitterest enemies, thus betraying friends and kin as well as country. But whereas a psychopath may have no concern for the feelings of others, he is still acutely aware of their perceptions. Alcibiades knew that a purple robe trailing in the dust would not have gone over well with the Spartans, nor would the gold and silver dishes that Alcibiades habitually ate off of in Athens. So he changed:

> People who saw him wearing his hair cut close, bathing in cold water, eating coarse meal, and dining on black broth, doubted, or rather could not believe, that he had ever had a cook in his house, or had ever seen a perfumer, or had worn a mantle of Milesian purple.[18]

He could change his public persona, but he was still Alcibiades, and he was soon up to his old tricks. He had an affair with the king of Sparta's wife, and when she became pregnant with his child, he bragged to all of Sparta that he had impregnated her so that his offspring would one day rule Sparta. Despite his callousness, the queen was so taken with Alcibiades that she privately called the child "Alcibiades." The king put Alcibiades on his to-be-assassinated list. It was time to move on.

The next stop was Persia, where Alcibiades betrayed the Spartans, of course, by urging the Persian king not to aid them in their war against Athens. The Persians had a different lifestyle from the Spartans, and once again Alcibiades reinvented himself. Plutarch notes that:

> At Sparta, he was devoted to athletic exercises, was frugal and reserved; in Ionia, luxurious, gay and indolent; in Thrace, always drinking; in Thessaly, ever on horseback; and when he lived with Tisephernes the Persian satrap, he exceeded the Persians themselves in magnificence and pomp.

He had, as it was observed, this peculiar talent and artifice for gaining men's affections, that he could at once comply with and really embrace and enter into their habits and ways of life, and change faster than the chameleon. One colour, indeed, they say the chameleon cannot assume: it cannot itself appear white; but Alcibiades, whether with good men or bad, could adapt himself to his company, and equally wear the appearance of virtue or vice.[19]

It is this gift for camouflage, this chameleon-like ability to take on whatever form would best suit his purposes, that defines the classic psychopath. Without that, he would be merely a scoundrel.

Eventually, Alcibiades made his way back to Athens where, incredibly, the people forgave his betrayals, welcomed him with open arms, and made him general once again. If all this is not enough to make Alcibiades the poster child for deception and psychopathy, consider this: This violent, brutal man who betrayed every country and nearly every person who ever befriended him, was Socrates's lover and arguably his favorite pupil. When Socrates eventually went on trial for his life, one of the accusations against him was that he had corrupted the youth of the city—and the example was Alcibiades.

I close Plutarch, and sit thinking about the implications of all this. I know all too well the research that finds that no treatment program has ever been successful with psychopaths. I just didn't know how early or how long people had been trying. But far from this being a question of Socrates corrupting Alcibiades, it was really a matter of Alcibiades being totally unchanged and unaffected by his long-term association with Socrates. This was, in fact, the first recorded example of treatment failure of a psychopath. If a giant like Socrates could not have an impact on Alcibiades, is it any wonder our cognitive behavioral treatment programs are floundering?

But still, Alcibiades will not leave me. I see him sometimes in my dreams, never on the dusty road to Sparta where he would transform himself by degrees—first the purple robe would go and then the hair cut close, until he arrived at Sparta so transformed the citizens compared him to Achilles. Nor do I see him returning to Athens triumphant from recent victories, the prodigal son trailing galleys and ornaments of the 200 ships he had sunk, returning to a hero's welcome, all past deaths and betrayals blinded by the sun shining on the enemy shields lying on his ships.

No, I see him before all that, before he left Athens in the first place. I see him at the defeat at Delium, riding behind Socrates. All around them the enemy was overtaking frightened Athenians who had dropped everything to run for their lives. All except Socrates. It was not Socrates's way to run from much of anything. Plato describes him at Delium as:

> Stalking like a pelican, and rolling his eyes, calmly contemplating enemies as well as friends, and making very intelligible to anybody, even from a distance, that whoever attacked him would be likely to meet with a stout resistance.[20]

Perhaps Socrates would have survived just on his fierce demeanor and on his fighting skills. Perhaps. But it did not hurt that he had the great Athenian general Alcibiades on horseback at his side. Although his horse would have carried him easily to safety, Alcibiades never left Socrates but instead stayed with him through the long retreat.

"Why?" I ask Alcibiades. "You were never loyal to anybody or anything. Why at Delium did you stand for Socrates?"

He tries to tell me he did it for love of his friend, but I don't believe him. Everything I know about psychopaths tells me it is not so, and yet. . . .

He wants his story to be told, I think, and someday I will write it. It is not just the story of Alcibiades, but a story of Socrates too, an odd man by standards then or now: the kind of man who might be walking at dawn and, seized by a line of thought, might stop on a street corner and stand there thinking for the next twenty-four hours while curious Athenians slept in the street through the night just to see how long he'd stay. Socrates never seemed to notice fatigue or cold and marched on ice with bare feet while others scrambled to make sure their own were well shod.

But Socrates was surely no saint in the way the world defines saints. When not fighting in one of Athen's frequent military excursions, he used his tongue as a sword, always to destroy—never to restore. It is no accident that Socrates is taught in law schools today and is credited with the invention of the cross-examination.

But whatever else he was—and I think of Socrates as neither a kind nor a compassionate man—he was no chameleon. He defied the Council of Thirty after they seized Athens, a very dangerous thing to do: The Council of Thirty was killing Athenians left and right for lesser insults. Socrates did it casually, without fanfare and with little regard for whether he lived or died. Whereas Alcibiades was whoever you wanted him to be, Socrates never bent with the wind nor tailored his presentation to any audience. If Alcibiades was a chameleon, a magician, a hologram of the viewer's projection, Socrates was the ultimate rock: unmovable and unchangeable. Blunt, proud, fearless, impossible to bribe or bully, he was, well, Socrates.

But who was this young man at his elbow? What did Socrates make of the golden boy with the impish smile, the winsome lisp, the retinue of admirers, the penchant for excess, the military brilliance, and the callous indifference to others? Was Socrates simply fooled by him? Not in the beginning. In the beginning Alcibiades tried to seduce Socrates by saying that he wished Socrates to "assist me in the way of virtue"[21] and offered to be his lover in exchange. Socrates replied:

> Alcibiades, my friend, you have indeed an elevated aim if what you say is true, and if there really is in me any power by which you may become better; truly you must see in me some rare beauty of a kind infinitely higher than any I see in you. And therefore, if you mean to share with me and to exchange beauty for beauty, you will have greatly the advantage of me; you will gain true beauty in exchange for appearance—like Diomede, gold in exchange for brass.[22]

But his mocking sarcasm did not last. Eventually Socrates succumbed to Alcibiades' charms. The chameleon found something that Socrates wanted to see.

It would be then a story of Socrates and Alcibiades. It is just like Alcibiades to be still clamoring for acclaim after 2,400 years. I will give him his due: He was a talented and courageous general who had a good military eye and who won a host of unlikely victories. Still, I don't think he will be entirely happy with the picture I paint. "You're making a mistake," I tell him. "I'm the wrong one for what you want. And besides, I know. I know why you stood for Socrates at Delium. It wasn't love at all. You always had an eye for quality. You could tell gold from brass, a good frieze from a bad one. You knew who he was, didn't you? You collected him like you would have a gold urn and protected him as carefully."

He never answers that.

I am sitting in a concrete box roughly six feet long and three feet wide. My claustrophobia is breaking in waves, and I wonder how anyone with even a touch of it survives a Supermax prison such as this one. I am waiting for a chameleon to open the door and walk into the room across from me. There is a glass wall between my room and his.

Somehow the Department of Corrections kept it out of the paper, a feat in this large northeastern state with its aggressive press, but the man in front of me compromised four correctional officers and a librarian in the medium security prison where he was housed, all at the same time. When he was finally caught, he had a bar in his cell and his own personal cell phone. He had drunk three-quarters of a bottle of vodka the night before and was having sex with the librarian on a regular basis.

The conning didn't stop when he was caught, of course. When he was transferred to Supermax, he had the local newspaper editor's home address within twenty-four hours of his arrival. There are no phone books in Supermax, so he must have persuaded a staff member to get the information for him, despite the fact that there was a sign on his cell saying that no staff member could talk to him alone. He wrote the newspaper editor who has been publishing editorials ever since on the unfairness of locking up this "innocent" man.

The records go on and on. He paid off a $9000 fine the court assessed with money he conned from strangers through the mail. While in Supermax, he persuaded a college student to cash her student loan check and send him all the money. As a result, she can't go to school this year and still has to pay off the loan. In fact, it turns out there are a number of women he's conned through the mail and even more he's seduced in person. His track record includes the seduction of a probation officer, a jailer, and a correctional officer's wife. He is very good at what he does.

I am thinking some combination of George Clooney and Brad Pitt is about to walk through the door. But I am wrong. A ordinary looking, tall, skinny kid with freckles walks in. "It is all technique," I realize. He seems almost nondescript; certainly he is not particularly good-looking.

He takes the few steps across the small room, puts both hands on the table and, unexpectedly, leans forward until his face is only a couple of inches from the glass. He stares at me without speaking. There is no expression at all on his face that I can read, and his pupils are dilated, so big in fact they dominate his face.

I am as taken aback as he intends me to be. I control my temptation to pull away and sit very still, saying nothing. He drinks me in, what I am wearing, the purse and the briefcase on the floor. I feel like I am being photographed, x-rayed really. What can he see? Long minutes pass, and then he sits down. The interview begins.

What was that all about? No doubt I *was* being photographed. He needs to know who I am to decide who he should be. It is a process he is always engaged in. Later I ask him, "If you were going to con and manipulate here in Supermax, how would you do it? How would you present yourself?"

He leans back and tilts his head thoughtfully. "Well," he says. "This prison is in a rural area. You have a lot of new staff here. A lot of staff who have never worked in corrections before. A lot of them haven't been too successful in sports or with women. I'd be the kind of guy they always wanted to be friends with in high school." I doubt Alcibiades himself could have done better.

As for what he got out of X-raying me? Nothing he liked, apparently. He sits through one interview but refuses to participate in the educational film I am making and does not want to talk with me again. I am apparently not looking enough like a potential victim these days. I just don't look quite lonely enough or depressed enough, or alternatively, hopeful and romantic enough. I don't look like I trust the world.

That still, small part of me that has been there for the last decade, that steady part is, I think, what he does not like. Not that he thinks he couldn't con me, only that he thinks it would take too much time. Not worth the investment.

It is very depressing to be unmasked so easily. I need a little dose of that chameleon thing, a lesson or two in camouflage. I stand in front of the mirror and try to look depressed or trusting or hopeful. I just look wary. Even a game fish will turn from a wary minnow when there are so many sweet, trusting minnows about.

When I come back another time, a correctional officer stops by to see me. A friend of his was one of those compromised at the previous prison. He has been bitter at Mr. Smith, the inmate; he was in charge of investigating his recent conning of women by mail. This time, however, it is a different story. He tells me Mr. Smith was so distressed after talking with me he almost threw up.

"Almost threw up?" I say, indignantly. "From what?"

"From remorse," he says, solemnly.

I look at him carefully, trying to figure out if he is serious. Finally, I say, "And what do you think of that?"

"Well," he tells me, "his behavior has changed. I monitor his mail, and his letters are different than when he first came."

I want to say something to him, although I don't. I want to say, "Tell me something. Does he remind you of somebody you wanted to be friends with in high school?"

Lord, protect us from the deceivers, for we cannot seem to protect ourselves.

8

Staff Seductions

It is perhaps not surprising that sexual predators who have never been arrested are so successful in fooling people. They simply take on the lifestyle and manner of genuinely nice people, and it is understandable, if tragic, that we can't tell the difference. It is more surprising that some predators with felony records find it so easy to get access to children. The information is there in the records, but even those who are supervising volunteer activities with children rarely check.

However, it is instructive to examine just how easy it is for offenders *currently* in prison to manipulate and seduce those with whom they come in contact. Every single staff member or volunteer who interacts with them knows they have done something possibly violent and always sufficiently illegal to warrant incarceration.

And yet, staff and volunteers are compromised every day in prisons. It would be difficult—I'd bet impossible—to find a prison anywhere in the world that has been operating more than two years that has not had to "walk staff out"; in other words, fire them for fraternizing, having sex with, or bringing in contraband for inmates. Inmates even seduce the general public through letters and phone calls to those outside the prison, as we saw in the offender's case in Chapter 7.

Staff seductions do not occur because guards and inmates are cut from the same cloth, as some like to claim. The ability of some inmates to compromise staff and others with whom they come into contact is, instead, an indicator of the power of the techniques they use.

Not every staff member or volunteer can be seduced, but given enough time and opportunity, the techniques offenders use will work on *somebody.*

Inmates get proficient, after a while, at predicting who will make a good target and who won't. They particularly like to target religious staff because they feel religious people are more trusting than others.

The problem is particularly acute in prisons, long-term mental hospitals, residential homes, and half-way houses where offenders and staff/volunteers spend long periods of time together. Such settings afford the offender time to target people, time to learn their vulnerabilities, time to build the right kind of relationship. The techniques they use can be clearly seen in such settings, but variations of them are run by psychopaths and sex offenders in any setting in which they operate.

For years I puzzled over how frequently staff and volunteer seductions took place, and I eventually obtained permission from a prison system to interview a series of men who had been successful in seducing more than one staff member each. One had seduced four female staff members, according to official records, but told me he'd "done seven." The warden blanched slightly when I reported this and protested the inmate was blowing smoke. But I am not so sure. We don't catch everybody for everything they do, and who would bet against a man who was caught for four?

What makes this man's case all the more remarkable is that he was not incarcerated for forging checks or tax evasion—an offense that could make a staff member tell him/herself that he is not physically dangerous. He is a triple murderer, a man who killed his own grandmother plus two boarders. It is not easy to see how he could announce to the world any more clearly that he is violent and not to be trusted. Nonetheless, his track record of seduction continues unabated: He is working on someone now, he tells me with a sly smile.

In trying to understand this phenomenon, I started by reading the records of these men. Of course, I couldn't rely on their word alone. As I expected, records indicated that the same techniques they used on staff, they also used outside the prison. Each of the men had long histories of conning family members out of money and support, convincing community members they were innocent, manipulating adults and children for sex, and in general conning anyone around them for whatever they wanted. No offender leaves his weapons of manipulation behind when he goes to prison: What they do outside, they do inside. And that is why I present them in this book, even though I will be talking here about the techniques they used in prison, and the offenders most people run into will be in the outside world.

For brevity, I will call all those seduced "staff members," although they were not always. They were sometimes staff, sometimes volunteers, sometimes community professionals who came into the prison once a week to lead a group or take a course, and sometimes members of religious groups who came in to counsel or convert.

In going through the records, it was striking how different these cases look from the offender's point of view as opposed to the staff member's. Take, for example, the young correctional officer who was caught having sex with an imprisoned gang member. She was fired and prosecuted but is still in love with the inmate, and she still writes him. He tells me the story from his point of view:

> As soon as she came, I know I had her. I was working out in the gym, and I winked at her. She smiled, and I thought, "I've got her."

Of course, the young officer did not know anything had begun, but the inmate knew what he was talking about. He played out his hand, flirting with her slowly and carefully, taking progressively more liberties. Finally one day he told her he wanted to write her a letter. She said, "I'll get in trouble for it." Wrong answer.

That's the problem in life. No warning music like in the movies. In real life, half the time you don't know you've given a stupid answer until it's too late. And it was a stupid answer because she said the letter would get *her* in trouble. As if he cared. The only response that would have stopped him cold was, "*You'll* get in trouble for it."

He replied simply, "Nobody would know." He continues his story:

> So I wrote her a letter. I told her I liked her a lot, and I thought she looked good. Nothing really sexual. "Don't let these people around you spoil you." I tried to make her think all these people

were racist. "Don't let them make you into a robot guard. Don't let them turn you."

It is a clever letter, and he had given considerable thought to it. He praised her appearance without saying anything overtly sexual. He also flattered her by implying she was different from others, better than the other guards who might "spoil" her. Finally, he played the race card.

Even so, he was gambling. Passing an officer a personal note is against prison rules. It was the one and only time in the process when he was vulnerable. He explains:

I have to give her something that she could lock you up for, and she doesn't do it. You got to take a risk. You got to gamble. If you don't gamble, you can't win.

Everything that happened from this point on would depend on her response to his letter. Ideally, from his point of view, she would write back. But that wasn't necessary. All he needed was for her not to turn the letter in. Not turning the letter in to prison officials would make her a co-conspirator and would also give him material for blackmail, should he need it later.

She kept the letter.

Who knows what this young and inexperienced officer thought? That it would all go away if she ignored it? That he sincerely liked her, and it would be a shame to get him in trouble for such a small thing? She didn't write him back. Did she think he would take a hint?

If we don't know her reasoning, we do know his reaction:

When she took the note, I had her. It's over. Really, she's in my control. I can basically do whatever I want. There's nothing you can do.

He continued the flirtation and eventually seduced her. "What would you have done," I ask, "if she had refused?" He answers:

I would have said "don't start anything with me you can't finish.

You're in a position to lose your livelihood, and I'm not. You've crossed the line. You're going to lose your livelihood."

The sexual contact that followed was eventually discovered, which was a disaster for the officer but not for the inmate. After all, he could now reap the status this liaison would bring him within the prison, and he couldn't do that until he was caught. Sure, he'd serve some time in segregation—a small price to pay. Another staff predator tells me:

Guys who get together with female staff are considered heroes in institutions. Not only are they getting what they want. They are getting the enemy to switch sides.

This inmate's status might have risen, but the officer's career, her relationships with other officers, her livelihood, and even her freedom were gone. She was fired and prosecuted for having sex with an inmate, all the while continuing to write to him. I ask him if he thought she cared for him. His reply:

She does. She does. She does. She thought she could control me bringing me things. But I own her. "I have information about you. I'm going to use it if you ever try to have control over me." She used to have control over me. Now I have control over her.

It is a fascinating response, most of all because I never asked him about control, only about caring. But he cannot answer a question about caring because he is psychopathic and does not know what it is. It is control he understands, and to him, that's what relationships are all about—who controls whom. He slips into a discussion of control within a single sentence of his response to a question about caring.

I do not mention any of this to him. I only ask him how he feels about her. He says:

She's a slut. She's a tramp. . . . They're all enemies to me. I don't care for her. . . . In the back of my mind she's a guard. She means nothing to me. I need to get everything I can from them as soon as I can before we get caught.

The harshness, the predatory tone of this statement gives me pause. I do not feel this way about animals. I do not even feel this way about anything. There are trees I care about more than that. She is not just less than human to him; she is less than a thing. It is particularly hard for me to imagine feeling such contempt for someone and then going to bed with him. And if I did, could I ever fool that person into thinking I loved him?

I sigh inwardly but keep my face carefully neutral. I know he will feed off almost any reaction I have. Alarm, disgust, anything of the sort will make him feel powerful and likely give him a high. After all, did he not agree to this interview just to brag about his cleverness?

This predatory view is pervasive among inmates who seduce staff and volunteers. One states:

Sometimes I see easy prey. Fuck her. She don't know me. I'm not looking for no love. I want some money. If she'll bring in some drugs, cool. If she'll have sex, better.

Yet another says:

If it doesn't result in a physical relationship, it may result in a TV, a pair of shoes, tapes, get something from them. It's a con.

I hear no remorse or guilt from these men. Staff seduction is a game. There is more joy in the winning than in the sex. Getting a staff member to bring in drugs is a better high than the drugs themselves. In any case, they justify it by telling me the staff bring it on themselves. As one explains:

I like living by my wits. The people who work here are slow. They're backwards. They're naïve. I just don't think they are smarter than me. We take advantage of them as much as we possibly can. They open themselves up to it.

Such inmates are confident, even grandiose about their chances of seducing staff. It is this confidence, I know, that has them talking to me. They feel they can outwit anyone:

> They're going to hang themselves. They think they know what they're doing. We've been playing this game a lot longer than they have. We have years and years of experience, and they don't. . . . You get good at it after a while if you do it all the time.

I sit and listen to these rambling tales of conquest, inmate after inmate, prison after prison. It is like listening to stories of a strange game and trying to deduce the rules and the strategies employed. The only guide I have is a book that twenty years ago described the sequence inmates go through when seducing staff.[1] As I put the pieces together, I decide nothing has changed. There is, indeed, a process that inmates go through when they seduce staff, one that eventually becomes automatic. The process is strikingly similar whether the inmate is in prison in Vermont or in California. It begins with obtaining information.

Obtaining Information

Talking with Staff

The process of gathering information starts the first day that new staff arrive. One offender describes it:

> You're new here. Someone would see you, how you carry yourself. How are you, Officer Salter? Seeing if you keep eye contact. What were you doing before you were here?

The last question is crucial. "If they'll talk about things outside the prison," inmates say about staff or volunteers, "they'll get personal." But getting personal is a long way off. The first step for inmates is watching, listening when staff talk to each other, simply showing an interest. The point is to find out problems, interests, vulnerabilities, hopes, anything that will provide material for future contacts.

Getting information, at least about some staff, does not seem to be that hard. Many offenders simply ask outright:

Find out something you're not supposed to know. What's her birthday? What kind of car? I'm having a conversation with her, but I'm collecting information from her that may be useful to me at a later time.

Behind the questions, the predatory intent lurks from the start:

She probably just thinks I'm being friendly, but I'm sizing her up. We're fattening them up for the kill.

It is not just female staff who are groomed or who reveal too much information. Men are compromised too, although more often to bring in contraband than to engage in sex. Still, the process of seduction and information gathering is the same. One inmate relates:

With men it's usually our age or younger. They talk too much. They tell us entirely too much information. They tell us what kind of bars they drink in.

Another offender tells me:

I can pretty much tell you which of the guards are drinking every night. Which ones are smoking dope. . . . People are who they are. They may put on some armor when they come through the door, but they can't not be who they are.

Something in me gets very still when he says this. It is that sound of "gospel truth" again. It is a worrisome statement. How can you keep people from being who they are?

Overhearing Staff Conversations

As fruitful as it is to talk directly with staff, inmates actually derive more information from overhearing staff talk to each other.

It is lunch time, and staff members are waiting in line in the inmate-run cafeteria. There are no inmates working there whom you know. While you wait, you talk to your friend about your child's problems in the fourth grade. The school has diagnosed him as having a learning disability and has been providing special tutoring. It's made all the difference. The inmate behind the counter appears to be paying no attention whatsoever.

Two months later, a different inmate comes to see you about his daughter, who is in the second grade, and the problems she's having in school. The school wants to test her, but he has refused. He doesn't think it will do any good, and he doesn't want her stigmatized. How tempting is it for you to mention that your son was also having problems and what a difference being tested and having special tutoring made? Will you even remember the conversation in the cafeteria line two months ago? Most likely not, and even if you did, would you be likely to associate that conversation with this one? Perhaps you are cautious and do not tell him of your own child, but does it make you feel more sympathetic toward this man because he has a problem similar to yours? Before you get too sympathetic, you'd better check and see if he even has a child.

This latter question is not academic. A prison psychologist reported providing grief counseling for weeks to an inmate who had lost a child. It ended when the counselor discovered the inmate had never had a child. This was years ago. He is now in a different prison, but recently, he heard another staff member talking about the grief counseling he was providing for an inmate who recently lost a child. The story sounded similar, and my colleague checked. Same inmate. And he still doesn't have a child.

Behavioral Observations

As easy as it appears to obtain information from talking to staff or from overhearing their conversations, words are not the only source of data.

Many inmates are better than most psychologists at behavioral observations. Consider this one:

> You can basically tell who's weak, who's going to make it in a penitentiary the first few weeks they're here. If they're not afraid of being off by themselves, they're going to be OK. If they're always hanging around someone, can't be by themselves, they're weak.

Signs of weakness will short-circuit the usual long-term "grooming" and cause inmates to move faster. For example:

> If guys see that, they'll go . . . I'm going to say something. She better not say something. She's scared.

The likelihood that staff members will be frightened varies from individual to individual and from prison system to prison system. In the rural state where these interviews took place, inmates reported less fear among the staff than in the larger penitentiaries in which some had also served time. Observes one:

> In this system they're not really afraid. They don't understand that they only go home because we let them. Because we choose to let them go home. That any time we wanted to, we could hurt one of them real bad.

The man who makes this statement looks directly at me when he says it. I keep my gaze flat and fight against recognition in my eyes. I know that he is talking about me right here in this room right now. He knows it too, but I don't think he knows I do. Inmates are often narcissistic and misogynistic. It is easy for him to believe I'm too stupid to know he's talking about me. And it is hard to intimidate people who don't recognize you're trying to intimidate them. Playing dumb is frequently the smartest thing to do. I keep my face steady and clueless. The moment passes; we move on.

What he says is true, of course. There are no guns allowed inside a prison. Officers, staff, even the warden walk daily among inmates without protection. The bars keep inmates from the outside world, but inmates lounge around day rooms, move between buildings, gather in the yards. It is the fear of consequences, not the lack of opportunity, that keeps them from attacking staff. Many things can override that fear: hate, psychopathy, a desire for revenge—even the thrill that a moment of power contains can do it.

Fear is a factor in a prison, but it is not the only factor inmates use to determine whom to target. There are other factors, even some that appear to be in the opposite direction. "She's action. She's action. She's action," one inmate says in describing a new female staff member.

"What does that mean?" I ask.

"You know. She acts loose, comfortable. Like she doesn't know it's a prison."

"What happens next?" I ask, "When someone is like that?"

"Then we say, 'She can be worked with. She can be worked with,' and the word will go down the line."

Damned if you're afraid. Damned if you're too comfortable. It's extremes, really, that inmates are looking for, anything that stands out from the norm. You're even damned if you're too strict. "Sometimes she's stern and shitty, and you just know," one predator says, a sentiment echoed by another:

> I've seen female officers with reputations for being a hard ass. Turned out she was one of the easiest to get to once you know.

From the moment any staff member walks into a prison, she or he is under scrutiny. The scrutiny is intense, professional, and organized. Inmates who decide a staff member is a possibility for seduction or compromise will pay other inmates to gather information for them. That information is rarely hard to come by. "You'd be amazed," one inmate tells me. "The inmate grapevine is huge."

Selecting a Target

The purpose of all of this information-gathering and behavioral analysis is just to select staff for further "grooming"—conning and manipulation. Few inmates are so narcissistic as to think they can manipulate everyone. More often the attitude is realistic. One states:

> The vulnerability—you can't just approach anyone. Because not everyone is going to fall for it. Not everyone is going to buy into what you have to say.

Vulnerability, however, is a broad concept, and once again, it is extremes that inmates are looking for. Divorce, financial problems, even the depressing impact of aging on women are all considered fair game. Almost any vulnerability will do. Consider this statement:

> With females, they normally prey on women who don't normally get the kind of attention that they're not exposed to outside the institution. When she comes in, they treat her like a queen. They don't joke about her weight. They don't make her feel stupid.

Because the information-gathering is so thorough, inmates know about problems that other staff members never consider they might know about. For example:

> There's a perfect one right here. Boyfriend/girlfriend where she has come in with black eyes, and he has been known to hit her on state property. . . . If going to him every night is a frightening experience and coming to work and talking to me every day is a pleasant experience, that's my in.

Of course, any kind of problem or vulnerability is considered fair game. If the staff member does drugs, it will not be a secret in a prison long. There are more experts on drugs inside prisons than in any other setting in the world. One offender says:

Eventually, something will let you know that he or she smokes weed. You start noticing them more. You start observing their actions. If you're a drug user, you tend to know the demeanor of a drug user, how they carry themselves.

But it is more than weaknesses or problems that define vulnerability for inmates. Staff who reach out and try to help inmates are considered possible targets. Religious staff are considered easiest to manipulate because, as one inmate says, "they look for the good in people," but any sort of caring is fair game.

"The reason I can be so successful," an inmate tells me, "is I find people who really care about other people." By his standards, he has, indeed, been successful. Because he has been frequently committed to mental health institutions, he has had access to female patients as well as staff. According to official records, he has at least twelve seductions of patients and staff to his credit, a tribute to his radar for finding both lonely and caring people.

The fact is, inside or outside, when vulnerability is found—be it loneliness or caring or religion—predators will certainly try to exploit it. As another offender says:

> If I see someone who I feel is vulnerable, I'm going to throw something out there. If I catch them, I'm going to run with it. If she's lonely or whatever, I'm going to try to capitalize on that. I'm going to use it to my advantage.

Tactics of Seduction: The Role of Reciprocity

After all the information-gathering and the selection of the most appropriate target, staff seductions begin, not by asking something from a staff member, but by giving something to them. Inmates intuitively recognize a social law called "reciprocity." It is a powerful principle of the social sciences and has been found in all cultures studied.[2] It is at work when the Hari Krishnas used to practically force a rose into your hands at an airport. Scientists who studied the Hari Krishnas—standing behind pillars in those same airports—say the average person frowned, walked a few steps, then dug in his or her pocket for change. Until they gave something back, they felt indebted. It is a powerful law, almost impossible for people to ignore or override.

Companies who send small amounts of money in exchange for filling in a questionnaire are using reciprocity. They know that those who cash the checks have a high rate of compliance. Those who don't fill in the questionnaire typically don't cash the checks. Nonprofits that send return address stickers in exchange for charitable contributions are using the same law. The American Disabled Veteran's Association, for instance, has discovered that they can increase their response rate to unsolicited mailings from 18 percent to 35 percent by including individualized address labels. Once the average person accepts something, he or she feels obligated to respond.[3]

The power of this law is hard to overestimate. In one study, just having a graduate student offer a soda to the participant of a research study doubled the number of raffle tickets the subject would buy after the study was supposedly over. And the irony, of course, was that each raffle ticket cost much more than the soda.[4]

What surprises me is that I did not know about this law and its power to affect behavior until I read the research on it, yet any staff predator in any prison knows it. Why does it take thirty years of research for the rest of us to understand phenomena that inmates grasp intuitively? It seems clear who the real experts are.

So what is it that offenders have to offer staff? For reciprocity to work, inmates must give first, ask later. But no staff member would simply take a gift from an inmate. That is against prison rules, and a gift too early in the process would almost surely be rejected. So what is it that gets in under the staff member's radar but nonetheless still triggers reciprocity?

The answer is, any number of things. It could be protection—or the myth of protection. Inmates will "offer to put you up on how things are run around the penitentiary, what inmates you should stay away from." Another describes the process:

You're new. You're in segregation. You don't know these guys from a can of paint. These guys are yelling all kinds of things. "Don't mind these guys. They're just restless."

To a new or insecure staff member, knowing when the situation is dangerous and when it isn't, who is dangerous and who is just noisy, is a valuable gift. Of course, the "protection" may be much more substantial than simply information or advice. The oldest con trick in the book is when one inmate threatens a staff member, and the "good" inmate rushes in to defend him or her. "Don't be bothering her," he will say. "Dr. X is the best psychologist here. She is the most professional member of the staff. She treats us right. Don't mess with her." The cigarettes he asks for later will often be the same ones used to pay off the "unruly" inmate.

Small favors are fair game too. They're not treating you right, an inmate may tell you, or "Your office is a mess. I got to clean the hall anyway. Why don't I do your office too? I got nothing but time."

But more than favors, more than protection, it is simply flattery that the inmate hands out lavishly. "You're not like the rest," they say. "You're the only one who can help." Like other parts of the process, this too is a conscious strategy on the inmate's part. One says:

The main thing is to stroke their ego. . . . If you can make a person feel good about themselves, most people will respond in kind. They will do things for you that are a little over the line, sometimes way over the line.

It isn't just praise that works. It is making the staff member feel efficacious. For example:

You can get almost anything you want if you let him think he's in control. "You're a white shirt. You can do whatever you want." Just make them feel powerful. First, get them to break little rules.

Consider the following exchange:

"Can I take a shower?" the inmate asks.

"It's after hours," the officer says. "You know that."

"You're the man," the inmate replies. "You say I can take a shower, I can take a shower."

Just make them feel powerful.

The Demand and the Lever

When the demand finally comes, it is after the information-gathering; after the selection of a specific target; after a campaign of giving praise, favors, even protection (or the illusion of it) to the staff member. It is after a campaign of bonding that starts by zeroing in on the staff member's interests, hobbies, even family problems. A personal relationship has been built, and the staff member has come to be in the offender's debt. The request for something back, when it first comes, will be for something so small as to seem insignificant, so tiny that refusing it would make the staff member feel petty. A surprising number of staff seductions start over a cigarette, extra pencils, even a French fry from a McDonald's bag. If you want someone to cross a line, it is important to make the line small—not a three-foot hurdle a staff member would have to leap, but just a pencil mark on the floor.

But if the request is small enough that the staff member doesn't sense the significance of this moment, the inmate does:

Got a bag from MacDonald's. "Hey man, give me some food."
He's crossed the boundary right now.

What starts as a French fry or a cigarette quickly escalates, although the initial request for illegal activity may still be polite. "Bring me some weed," the inmate may say smiling. "You told me you get high. Let me see what you've got going out there."

Sooner or later it becomes considerably less polite. "Bring me some weed or don't bring your ass back to work." It's the same request, just at a different point in the process.

As the demands escalate, the staff member may balk, and if so, the lever will be brought out. That too may be something small initially, perhaps fruit from the "innocent" conversations the staff member has had with the inmate.

> I know this and this and this. . . . I know all kinds of personal business about her. I know her father sexually abused her and all that.

Personal information may seem like a small thing to use for blackmail, but it is often enough. The information is proof of a personal relationship between inmate and staff. It is proof, at the least, that the staff member has been foolish and stands to lose face with the other officers if it is discovered. The content may be tender as well. Has the staff member told her family that her father sexually abused her as a child? Does her mother even know? Does she want the whole staff and all the inmates at the prison to know?

If the staff member doesn't balk, the hooks will soon be in too deep to get free. From then on, life only gets grimmer. One offender reports:

> They've got their hooks in you, and as long as you don't want to lose your job, you don't want to go to jail for supplying drugs, as long as you don't want the shame, you're going to do what you're asked—actually, told. You're not actually asked anything.

The demands will continue and may even escalate. An inmate who was running several staff members at the same time tells me the whole thing got out of hand:

> I enjoyed it so much I abused it. It got to the point every day I wanted something. I felt free in a way.

Eventually, at least in some cases, the relationship is discovered and the staff member fired and often prosecuted. She/he has lost her or his job, colleagues, livelihood, and any hope of continuing with a career in corrections. None of that was of any concern to the inmates who sat across from me. Instead, they had an unmistakable air of glee in describing their cleverness.

But there was one surprise left. I have been routinely surprised in the course of these interviews: surprised about how predatory the process is, surprised at the role of reciprocity. Yet I can hardly believe my ears when an inmate says he asked a psychologist in the prison about me: "She said you were a really nice person, and you were very professional." I look down at my notes on how inmates use praise to seduce staff.

Another inmate in a different interview leans back, puts his hands behind his head, and says casually, "So, why do you make educational films?"

"I like to make educational films," I say carefully.

"Yea, but why about this?" he asks. "Why not something else?"

He says this after he has just told me the importance of getting personal information from staff. "If they'll talk about something outside the prison," he has said, "they'll get personal." Revealing his method doesn't even slow him down from trying to pull the same thing on me.

Thoughts go through my head. What I really want to do is yell, "Give me a break. You spend three hours telling me how you get staff to talk about things outside the prison and then you try to pull the same thing on me *in the same session*? Hello. What do you think? I'm a potted plant? Hubris, hubris, hubris. Wait a week."

I do not say it. I smile politely and say softly, "I appreciate your offer of a demonstration, Mr. Smith. Can't take you up on it, but I do appreciate it."

Then I go home and write mysteries where an impulsive protagonist yells, "Hubris, hubris, hubris. Wait a week."

9

Rose-Colored
Glasses and Trauma

A neighbor sits in my kitchen. "I choose to believe there is good in everyone," she tells me, "because of the unintended consequences to my life if I do not. I feel an openness to others that wouldn't be there if I didn't believe that there's good in everybody."

I like this woman a great deal, and I worry for her. What she is saying sounds naïve to me, and worse, dangerous. But this woman is neither naïve nor foolish. She is, in fact, one of those people of whom the world needs more. She goes to medical school half-time so that she can be more present for her family. She is an outstanding parent, a gentle and responsible person, an altogether constructive force in the world. She does not think salvation lies in a bigger VCR or a new DVD. As a result, her children have grown up without the mall-hunger that eats into the souls of so many. Instead, they are responsible and self-assured. Each spring, her family goes to Haiti so she and her husband can volunteer in the health clinics. She wants her children to see the larger world and all that must be done before everyone has a roof over his or her head.

What do I say to this woman? Nothing I can say will change her outlook and, actually, it's working pretty well. If her beliefs allow her to function this well, shouldn't I be saying, as the woman did in the *When Harry Met Sally* restaurant scene, "I'll have what she's having?" I'm silent for a moment, thinking that anything I say will make me sound like the Grinch Who Stole Christmas.

Finally, I decide I respect this woman too much to be evasive. Shutting up means closing up, and I would like to expand my dialogue with her, not strangle it by not being present. And then again, it is also true she peels back the skin on cadavers and dissects the muscles. As if anything I could say would shake her.

So I answer honestly, the backlog of interviews with rapists, child molesters, sadists, and psychopaths jangling like discordant bells in my head. "You'd be lunch," I say, "in a prison environment. The psychopaths would see you coming. And they would very quickly figure out what you want to see and give it to you. Before you know it, they'd be talking about spiritual values and poverty around the world." The problem is, of course—and we both know it—the types of people who exist in prison also exist outside of prison. People run into psychopaths every day, and I am thinking that sooner or later, she may also.

"To me," I say, "you sound like a minnow arguing there aren't any bass in the world. You believe what you want to be true. What you're really doing is projecting who you are out there. But there are people out there who are very different from you.

"Not to mention it's a moot point," I go on, "as to whether there is good deep down in everybody because there are some folks where you and I are never going to find it."

She laughs. The fading sun lays ribbons of light across the blue table top in my kitchen. Vapor rises from her tea. What I'm saying sounds surreal here, belied by the murmur of children's voices in the play room, the sound of jazz, the smell of wood burning in the fire place. In this easy moment, the joy that is never far from the surface of her face lies open and exposed. The wariness that is never far from the surface of mine is banked. I think the world I've built in this small, comfortable home is a bubble that I will protect with tooth and claw. She feels the world she has created in her own loving home is a mirror of the larger world. She would reason with an intruder. I would shoot him.

Do we live in the same world? Yes and no. What world each of us lives in has as much to do with our beliefs as it does with the facts in front of us. The facts are always swept up in theory, in our beliefs about the meaning of what we see. My neighbor and I both see assault and suffering in the world. We just don't draw the same conclusions from it. I will argue here that one's worldview is a complex and paradoxical issue. The most optimistic viewpoints on the world can be shown to make us healthier and happier, but also can—unchecked—make us vulnerable to predators as well. But how and where and when to scan those around us for predators as opposed to looking for the good in everyone are not easy questions to answer.

People want to make the world have meaning, but the randomness of trauma defies meaning. Malevolence defeats it. *When Bad Things Happen to Good People* is a book that tries to make sense of the fact that dreadful things happen for no good reason. It was a best-seller when it was published twenty years ago, and it is still in print today. Why is this book so successful? Because it tries to make sense of something that most people find senseless and unnerving, the randomness of trauma.

It is a curious phenomenon, this need to find meaning, even justice and purpose, in the random events that afflict humankind. After all, logic would question the notion that there is any meaning to be found. Why shouldn't bad things happen to good people? What reason is there to think that smallpox or brain tumors select on the basis of virtue or vice?

What the success of *When Bad Things Happen* and countless other books on the same topic demonstrates is that the meaning that seems most comforting to people has a distinct rose-colored look to it. I would argue—and the research would concur—that almost everyone lives with illusions that make the world less frightening. Most often, these illusions imply that diseases, hurricanes, faulty brakes, and nuclear bombs are moral entities that are sensitive to issues of justice. Alternatively, some believe that such disasters are tools in the hands of a higher power, which uses them selectively and with discretion. But what kind of a higher power would use smallpox? Nobody you'd want to meet, that's for sure.

These illusions have their pros and cons. Once I was hiking in the Sierras and came across a giant sign at the entrance to a trail. The sign said, "The Mountains Don't Care." The rangers, it seemed, had had enough of hikers who ventured up to commune with Mother Nature without ice axes, warm coats, or water. Lost in the glory of the mountains, they would trust the Great Spirit to take care of them. But the Sierras obey their own gods, ones that have to do with wind and temperature and altitude. The temperature can slide like a bobsledder on a record run, and spring days that begin with sweat and suntan lotion can end with whiteouts and frostbite. Too many people have died in T-shirts, curled up in snow banks, with no idea even which way leads home. What concern is it to the mountains whether these two-legged ants live or die?

Why do bad things happen to good people? Because the mountains don't care. But we so badly want them to.

The great gift of consciousness, of course, is that you don't have to live with what's "out there" in the "real world." The mountains may not care, but we are free to believe they do. In the "real world" we live in—the one inside our heads—the dialogue goes on endlessly between what's out there and what we *want* to be out there. All truces in this endless war are transient, all settlements subject to later interpretation. "Things as they are/Are changed upon the blue guitar," Wallace Stevens wrote. And then he warned us, "I cannot bring a world quite round,/Although I patch it as I can."[1]

Of course, he lies. Stevens brings the world round quite nicely, as all the great poets do, but then again, if it's a question of just taking the rough edges off reality, you and I are as gifted as he. A vast body of research confirms my suspicion that my friend's rose-colored point of view is more common than my more cynical one.[2] In fact, as early as 1978, there were more than one thousand articles on what are termed "positive illusions," the tendency of people to soften the world, ignoring and minimizing its bad aspects and overgeneralizing its good ones—and the research has only picked up speed since then. In general, people hold positive illusions about themselves, about the amount of control they have over their fates, and about the benevolence of the world. I will look at each of these in turn. As will be seen, these positive illusions have an impact on our functioning (mostly pro) and on our susceptibility to predators (mostly con). Finally, these illusions are themselves susceptible to the impact of trauma, which sometimes shatters them, leaving a bleak world in its wake.

Self-Regard: The Average Person Is Better Than the Average Person

Most people evaluate themselves positively. In fact, just about everybody seems to feel that he or she is above average on a wide variety of traits and attributes, for instance, happiness, say, or driving ability.[3] In one study, 87 percent of the participants rated themselves more positively than the average peer of the same age and gender.[4]

In addition, when asked to rate their current mood over the period of a month compared to *their own typical mood state,* almost all the people in one study rated themselves as happier at that moment than they *themselves* typically were. In short, everybody is not only happier than the average person; people are happier than they, themselves, typically are.[5]

Of course, the above-average ratings only extend to *positive* personality traits. Most people think they are below average on negative traits.[6] In any case, any trait they don't score well on, people decide is not that important.[7] One's strengths are viewed as important and rare; one's failings, unimportant and common.[8]

Unfortunately, this undue sense of competence and confidence also translates into a belief that we can detect deception better than we actually can. In reality, people are pretty lousy at telling who's lying, a finding supported through twenty years of research.[9] In the typical experiment, subjects are given audio- or videotaped interviews and asked to say whether each person is lying or telling the truth. Accuracy is almost never above 60 percent, not much better than flipping a coin. Some groups do worse than chance (i.e., they would be better off flipping a coin).

Although much of this research has been conducted on college students, it has also been replicated on professional groups that have considerable experience with deception.[10] For example, some researchers have found that customs inspectors were no more accurate than college students in spotting lies.[11] Others found no difference between federal law enforcement officers and college students in detecting lies, regardless of their level of experience,[12] whereas still others found that police officers performed no better than chance.[13] Paul Ekman, likely the world's foremost expert on deception, studied U.S. Secret Service, federal polygraphers, judges, police, psychiatrists, and students on their ability to spot lies.[14] None of the groups did well. The Secret Service did better than other groups, but only 29 percent were able to detect deception at above-chance levels.[15] Only 12 percent of psychiatrists were accurate. In general, the groups performed at chance levels; once again, they might just as well have flipped a coin.

"A man's gotta know his limitations," Dirty Harry said, but it seems we don't. In one study, federal law enforcement officers were more confident than college students about their ability to detect deception, but, nonetheless, they were no more accurate, which is to say, not accurate at all.[16] Others have also failed to find a relationship between confidence and accuracy.[17] For example, Ekman found that confidence was unrelated to accuracy for most of his groups with two exceptions: federal officers and Secret Service agents.[18] But the findings weren't straightforward; in fact, they were odd and disturbing. It turned out that federal officers weren't bad at knowing how accurate they were likely to be before they did the experiment. Their confidence in how well they did afterward, however, had nothing to do with how well they really did.

The findings in regard to Secret Service agents were even more puzzling. There was no correlation between their confidence and how well they did before they took the test. After they took the test, they were dead wrong about how accurate they had been. The ones who were the least accurate thought they were the most.

And these are the pros.

When all the group findings from Ekman's study were put together, nothing, not sex, age, or years of job experience, made any difference in accuracy. However, there were two particularly unusual findings when the data were analyzed by occupational group: Both Secret Service agents and polygraphers got *less* accurate as they got older. All of the Secret Service officers and the polygraphers who scored at better-than-chance levels were under the age of forty. Also, for the Secret Service group, the more years of job experience, the less accurate they were.

I cannot explain these findings. It doesn't surprise me that people are less accurate than they think they are or that confidence has nothing to do with accuracy. But I am truly mystified as to why more age and more experience would translate into less accuracy. It is possible that the age findings are related to the fact that successful lie detectors pay more attention to body language than to words, and the ability to read nonverbal signals could diminish with age. But that is only speculation.

Having Too Few Doubts

Among the positive illusions we must monitor is our bias toward believing what people tell us.[19] Over and over, research shows that the default option is to believe what we hear and what we read. And it doesn't take much to even increase that bias further. Simple things such as repeating a false assertion will increase the chances that people will believe it.[20] There are even studies that show people will believe statements that are openly labeled false under certain circumstances.[21]

This propensity to believe almost anything is so striking in the research that it has revived the old Spinoza/Descartes disagreement. Benedict de Spinoza held that comprehending and believing were the same thing, that one cannot comprehend a proposition without believing it. René Descartes wrote that people understand a proposition and then make a decision about whether to believe it or not—a position that seems intuitively true. However, if Spinoza's view sounds incredible, consider an analogy with perception. If you see a tree, you accept it as real. Under certain circumstances you may later decide it is a mirage, but that is after the fact; in general, seeing is believing.

There is no obvious reason to assume that verbal propositions work the same way, but assumptions aside, they may. There is an increasing amount of research to show that people immediately, automatically, and unconsciously assume statements are true, and only afterward do they evaluate them for possible falsehood. If they then decide the statements are false, they have to unlearn them, a process that does not occur if they are distracted in the evaluation process.

For example, Dr. Daniel Gilbert and colleagues have shown that just having subjects count numbers imbedded in the text of statements labeled "true" or "false" increases the chance that statements labeled "false" will be remembered as "true" while not changing memory of the "true" statements at all.[22] They argue that this would only happen if the default option in our brains was set to "true" and the subsequent reevaluation to "false" required time for us to reconsider, time that wasn't there if the subject was too busy counting numbers.

If it seems hard to see the relevance of this process to sexual predators and deception, consider Gavin De Becker's work on predators.[23] One of the main mechanisms predators use when approaching strangers is to talk a lot and to give unnecessary detail, often about topics unrelated to the exchange. For instance, De Becker describes a young woman carrying heavy groceries up the stairs to her apartment. Several cans of cat food fell out of a bag and rolled down the stairs. Immediately, a man she had not seen when she came in picked them up and brought them to her. He offered to carry her bags for her and lightly ridiculed her caution when she was reluctant. Once he had the bags, he proceeded to chat all the way up the stairs about a cat he once forgot to feed for a friend. Too much detail, De Becker says. Too much distraction, the research would add.

Finally, at the top of the stairs, she was hesitant to let this stranger carry the groceries into her apartment. "Hey, we can leave the door open like ladies do in old movies. I'll just put this stuff down and go. I promise," the affable stranger said.[24] If someone promises you something you didn't ask them to promise, De Becker notes, assume they will do the opposite. Very true. But in addition, I would add, if someone distracts you immediately after meeting them, assume there is a reason—particularly if the setting is isolated. Distraction keeps people from evaluating the encounter and from considering whether the statements and the presentation may be false.

The purpose of all that gabbing on the stairs was to distract the young woman from the realization that she had seen no one at the bottom of the stairs when she came in, that the door to the building had not opened since she entered, and that none of the apartment doors had opened either. So where had he come from? He had to have been hiding in the stairwell when she went by. Had she known that, she might not have been so willing to give him her groceries or to let him into her apartment. She might have made an excuse to go back downstairs and "retrieve" something she left. Had she not been distracted, she might not have spent the next three hours being raped, assaulted, and nearly killed.

Women, it seems, are more vulnerable either to believing or to pretending to believe than men. This is unfortunate because the majority of sexual assaults are against women and girls, and they are precisely the population for whom gullibility is most dangerous. But research on men and women and the detection of nonverbal clues has shown a strange pattern. Women are normally much better than men at reading facial clues and identifying emotion—unless you're talking about hidden emotion.

When it comes to hidden emotion, men get better the more the real emotion "leaks" through tone of voice or gesture—hardly a surprising finding. The more obvious the discrepancy between what the person says and their body language, the more the men pick up on it.[25] But how to explain that the more discrepant the nonverbal and verbal messages become, the *less* women read hidden emotion. And this from a population that is better than men in reading emotion in general.

Scholars debate why women do not apply their skills to masked emotion, especially when the hidden emotion becomes more and more obvious. The consensus seems to be that it is not because of an *inability* to read the clues—women have demonstrated their skills to do so—but rather that it is due to an *unwillingness* to do so. Calling attention to discrepancies would break the social contract. It might be considered rude. Indeed, it could be considered eavesdropping.[26] Instead, women are motivated to smooth over conflicts, a tendency some consider a strength. The researcher Judith Hall has been quoted as saying:

> Women are just doing something that represents an intelligent social strategy. Smooth interaction requires that people not notice or comment on every little lapse in decorum, or every little bit of insincerity. Social life works by ignoring little social lies. Women seem wiser to this than men.[27]

Maybe so. But what is a strength in one setting may be a vulnerability in another. If ignoring emotional leakage that suggests deception is a kindness in dealing with social lies, it is a different matter altogether in dealing with a stranger who smiles with his mouth and not with his eyes.

My point is simply that one reason people are vulnerable to predators is because we think we can detect liars better than we actually can. In actuality, we generally believe what we're told or what we read. Women, particularly, seem to ignore signs of insincerity in others in favor of maintaining smooth social functioning.

But our confidence in our ability to detect lying is going to be hard to change, partially because it is part of a larger issue. It is part of an inflated self-image that traditional psychology might call narcissism but that turns out to be entirely normal. We think we are better at many things than we are, and most of the time, those beliefs serve us well. Our belief in ourselves, our hopefulness, and our confidence in our abilities are normally strengths, and as will be shown, they make us healthier physically and mentally. But it is not just our views of our own efficacy that are slanted in a positive way. Our beliefs regarding how much control we have over our own fates and how benign the world is are biased as well. Both of those beliefs affect our ability to protect ourselves and affect our treatment of victims of trauma.

Personal Control over Events

We would all like to be masters of our fate, and often we pretend we are, even when we aren't. People, at least in the Western hemisphere, tend to think they can control even chance events. Gamblers have been known to throw the dice softly for low numbers and hard for high numbers. Some require silence to throw so they can concentrate more.[28]

Likewise, legions of players, coaches, and fans continue wearing whatever article of clothing they had on when their team won a big game. True, sports have more to do with skill than craps, and one can argue that whatever makes a player or coach feel confident may affect the result. Still, it isn't clear that a fan sitting in front of a TV wearing his Green Bay Packers cap is likely to actually have much of an impact.

We treasure the illusion of control even when there is no logic at all to our beliefs. People will bet less in a game of chance against a confident opponent than one who appears meek and ineffective. They have more confidence in a lottery card they have chosen for themselves than one that is chosen for them, and they are resistant to trading one they have chosen for themselves for one that has better odds of winning.[29]

The truth is that people's minds turn from the notion of random. We don't seem to like it any more than Albert Einstein did when he rejected the notion of randomness in physics by saying, "God does not play dice with the universe."

Unfortunately, this same belief in personal control means that people are often less than kind to victims of assault. At 10:30 in the morning one summer day in 1990, an American woman named Susan Brison went for a walk down a sunny, country road in a village outside Grenoble, France.[30] She was quite suddenly attacked from behind, sexually assaulted, and strangled unconscious, eventually several times. She awoke from the last strangulation attempt in time to see her attacker swinging a large rock toward her head. Later she regained consciousness and crawled out of the ravine where he had left what he thought was her corpse. She spent eleven days in the hospital, the first of them trying to survive.

It is hard to imagine how anyone could have blamed this woman for this assault. In fact, given the circumstances and her condition, neither the police nor the hospital personnel ever even entertained the possibility. She was, after all, in what was thought to be a safe area, in the middle of the day, wearing baggy pants and a sweat shirt.[31] She did not trust a stranger; she was not even fooled, she was attacked from behind. What could this woman have even done differently, except perhaps cower fearfully in her room on a bright summer day?

Nonetheless, when she later spoke with a victim's assistance coordinator regarding legal advice, she was told that the counselor herself had never been a victim, and that Dr. Brison might benefit from the experience by learning not to be so trusting of people and not to go out late at night. She gave Dr. Brison no chance to remind her that she had been attacked suddenly, from behind, in the middle of the morning.

The counselor's response was not an isolated phenomenon. Once, I was training in a civil commitment center for sex offenders. In fifteen states, at the time of this writing, sex offenders who have served their prison sentences can, under certain conditions, be civilly committed to a secure setting for an indefinite period of time after their incarceration expires, until they are supposedly successfully treated. Typically, the top 10 percent of high-risk sex offenders (or less) are retained.

At that training, I was showing a video of a man who answered an ad for a motorcycle for sale. Finding a woman home alone with only her baby, he waited until she turned around to pull the cover off the motorcycle, then jumped her. He wrestled her to the ground and then put a knife to her throat and forced her inside the house. In the lengthy assault that followed, he told her at one point to put her baby to bed in the next room.

Three different women that day, women who worked in this center for sexual offenders, got angry at the woman for not taking her baby and escaping through the window when he told her to put him to bed. Of course, the victim had to contend with a knife-wielding rapist in the next room, which was less than fifteen feet away, who would clearly have heard the noise. None of us knew how securely the window was fastened or what it would have taken to get through it. None even knew whether it was the type that could be opened. None of us knew if it was even on the first floor of the house. None of us should have been judging her, given we were not the ones with a baby in our arms and a rapist with a knife in the next room.

I was taken aback by their hostility to this woman, whom they blamed for not escaping from the assault, until I began to think how the world might look from the standpoint of women who work with high-risk, very assaultive sex offenders. Maybe, just maybe, it becomes very important for a woman in that situation to believe that she can control her fate, that nothing like that could happen to her. But buying a sense of safety in that way is a two-edged sword: It may make us feel safer and more secure, but it adds to the distress of those already victimized. We retain our peace of mind by making victims pay for it.

But it is not just onlookers who blame victims for assault, it is often the victims themselves. It is disconcerting for clinicians to hear a woman say she should have known better than to cut across the arboretum at noon or to walk around a local pond at 3:00 in the afternoon. Women decide the skirt they were wearing was too short or their hair too long. They believe they should have taken the elevator rather than the stairs or the stairs rather than the elevator. It doesn't always make sense, and it pains others listening to it. Maybe, just maybe, others think, the rapist had some responsibility here, not this poor woman walking across campus in the middle of the day.

On the other hand, what would you rather believe? That you could change the length of your skirt or your hair and never be raped again? Or that it was a random assault, which nothing you did or could do would have prevented, and therefore, could happen again at any time, any place, for the rest of your life? Not surprisingly, a study found that the victims who were most psychologically distressed following rape were those who had been following their personal rules of safety at the time.[32] I would suspect there was nothing else they knew to do, and the realization of their ongoing vulnerability could not be avoided.

Even Brison, the American woman attacked in the French village, has cut her hair short in hopes she could be mistaken for a man from behind. She did this knowing full well it would not have prevented the assault she endured. A man she saw casually standing in his front yard that summer day—a man who saw her from the front—was the one who waited until she passed, followed her, and then attacked her from behind.

"From the car to the house. From the house to the car," an offender once said to me in an interview. "You have no idea how vulnerable you are." And I thought of all those times to come, walking from the house to the car, from the car to the house, and wanted to find some way to deny what he said. Perhaps if I changed the length of my skirt. Or wore my hair shorter.

The World Is a Pretty Nifty Place

Listen to New Age philosophy, and you will discover a remarkable thing: It consists almost entirely of beliefs that the world is controllable and benign. We all have a guardian angel who looks after us. Everything happens for a reason. The bad things that happen in our lives are all simply there to teach us karmic lessons. This is surely the best of all possible worlds. In fact, we really don't have any problems at all that can't be cured by tuning into a higher energy level.

If you think this latter must be an exaggeration, read *There's a Spiritual Solution to Every Problem* by the best-selling author Wayne Dyer.[33] The book begins with two quotes, "You have no problems, though you think you have" (from "A Course in Miracles") and "There is nothing wrong with God's creation. Mystery and suffering only exist in the mind" (from "Ramana Maharshi"). "If God is good and God made everything, then everything is good," Dyer tells us.[34]

But how do I tell that to my clients who were raped and molested as children, those who have been the victims of domestic violence, and most of all, those who have had children abducted or murdered? Do I really tell them that they are simply vibrating at the wrong frequency, as Dyer contends, that illness, fear, and anxiety occur when people are vibrating at 10,000 cycles per second? If they could just get up to the 100,000 cycles per second, they'd be in the region of sound, light, and spirit, in Dyer's opinion, and pretty much in orbit, in mine.

What is billed as "New Age" is really older than time. People have always wanted to feel safe in the world and to fend off the frightening reality that the death rate is one per person and that the timing of it appears to have nothing to do with goodness. The writer Ann Lamott warned against "spiritualizing your hysteria,"[35] but she was up against a tidal wave. We all spiritualize our hysteria. The truth is hard to live with: The world is actually a pretty dicey place. A lot of bad things can happen out there, and often do.

Answer these questions before you read further. What is the probability that you will be in a fire serious enough to cause injury or property damage in your lifetime? What are the chances you'll be robbed or be in a car wreck serious enough to cause injury? What are the chances that a loved one of yours will die from suicide, homicide, or accident? If you live in the United States, and you came up with single digit answers, you are kidding yourself.

In 1992, for example, Dr. Fran Norris published a study of the frequency of trauma in a U.S. sample.[36] Table 9.1 shows the results.[37]

TABLE 9.1   Lifetime Exposure to Trauma in Four U.S. Cities

Type of Trauma	Percentage Exposed Lifetime
Fire[1]	11
Physical Assault	15
Robbery	25
Motor Vehicle Crash[2]	23
Loved One Lost from Homicide, Suicide or Accident	30
Some Kind of Trauma	69

[1]Serious enough that injury or property damage occurred.
[2]Serious enough that someone was injured.

Sixty-nine percent of us will suffer some significant trauma in our lifetime—and those are external accidents and hazards alone, not including heart disease, cancer, and every other catastrophic illness. Thirty percent of us will lose a loved one to homicide, suicide, or accident. That's one in three.

"That it's rough out there and chancy is no surprise. Every live thing is a survivor on a kind of extended emergency bivouac," Annie Dillard wrote[38] in a sentence that startled me. Although we'd probably agree that ladybugs and night crawlers live in such uncertainty, or even people in the Middle Ages, it's a surprise to most of us that we do too. We stay deliberately unaware of the odds on this slot machine we play.

The need to view the world positively runs deep. It is found in our language and even in what material we find easy to learn and what we have trouble remembering. Consider these findings from one of the original summaries of the literature, *The Pollyanna Principle: Selectivity in Language, Memory, and Thought*:

1. When exposed to pleasant and unpleasant experiences for equal periods of time, people report the pleasant were more frequent.
2. People remember pleasant information better and more accurately than unpleasant.
3. Pleasant information is easier to learn than unpleasant.
4. People recognize pleasant words quicker than unpleasant.

5. People exaggerate the likelihood of pleasant events. For example, in one experiment, positive outcomes whose true probability was 10% were judged as only slightly less likely to occur than negative outcomes whose probability was 90%.

6. The pleasant member of antonym pairs is said before the unpleasant, for instance, good-bad, sweet-sour, right-wrong.

7. Pleasant words tended to enter the English language first and have higher frequencies than do unpleasant.

8. People use positive terms far more often than negative whether in writing or speaking.

9. People slant their memories in a positive direction over time. For example, years later mothers reported that their children walked earlier, slept better, ate better and were toilet trained more readily than records indicated they had reported at the time. Indeed, the children also were happier, easier and sucked their thumbs less in memory than they had in reality.

10. People think the present is better for them personally than the past and the future will be better still regardless of the actual probabilities. For example, in a study of 145 high school girls, 1/2 thought they would marry wealthy men soon after graduation and live happily ever after. The other half thought they would have high paying glamorous jobs by the time they were twenty-five. In reality, in their area only 4 out of 10 could be expected to earn salaries above the poverty level, only 3 out of 10 would finish college, and 4 out of 10 would be divorced or widowed.[39]

This deep bias toward the positive in memory, thought, and speech acts as a filter. No wonder we think the world is benign and most of what happens is good—if that is what we selectively remember. The exception is that people who are depressed do not, of course, see the world nearly as positively, but then again, they are depressed.

But you might well ask, what of the news? On any given day the news is uniformly negative. If there is anything good happening in the world, the major newspapers and TV stations manage not to report it.

Authors Margaret Matlin and Daniel Stang had an answer for the popularity of the news. They found there was a competing tendency to focus on the novel, and because good news is considered routine, bad news is the exception. But, unfortunately, bad news is not as much of an exception as we would like to believe.

A Just World

When we are confronted with bad news, it seems we try desperately to make sense of it, to put it in some framework that allows us to explain, even to rationalize it, while maintaining our overall positive worldview. Most of all, it seems, we want to believe the outcome is just.

A researcher and teacher named Melvin Lerner first framed the notion of "a just world."[40] He had once taught medical students in a state with large mining regions. As part of their training, he had the task of introducing them to the impact of poverty on health care: for example, poor housing, hygiene, nutrition, and the like. Even though the extensive poverty in that state was undeniably due to circumstances beyond the workers' control—demand for coal had gone down, mines had been automated, and unemployment had soared—nonetheless the students blamed the victims.

> Typically, very early in that kind of presentation, one of the students would let me know that he grew up with "those people," and I didn't know what the hell I was talking about. Those people were happy living like that. They were just the kind of folks who would cheat and connive and let their kids go hungry rather than go out and get a decent job. There was plenty of work for everyone if they just wanted it—if they'd just go out and look for it. No one had to go hungry. They were lazy, irresponsible.[41]

To his credit, Lerner did not simply stereotype the staff or medical students that he worked with by labeling them "insensitive" or "callous." He asked himself the question instead of why staff and students were reacting that way.

And thus began a program of research that culminated in a book called *The Belief in a Just World,* which he subtitled *A Fundamental Delusion.* The research showed time and again that people blamed others for whatever outcome occurred, regardless of whether there was any logical relationship between the behavior and the outcome. Even when the students were told the outcome was randomly assigned, they still rated victims lower on a variety of traits and characteristics than they did others in the same experiments who they were told were randomly selected to have a better outcome.

How does this apply to predators? It applies because over and over victims are blamed for their assaults. And when we imply that victims bring on their own fates—whether to make ourselves feel more efficacious or to make the world seem just—we keep ourselves from taking the precautions we need to take in order to protect ourselves. Why take precautions? We deny the trauma could have easily happened to us. And we also hurt people already traumatized. Victims are often already full of self-doubt, and we make recovery harder by laying inappropriate blame on them.

In the Chowchilla kidnapping case (discussed below), for example, a case in which an entire school bus of children was kidnapped and (temporarily) buried alive, one mother who attended church regularly and whose child was dropped off the bus before the kidnapping occurred, explained her daughter's near miss by saying, "The Lord is faithful to those who are faithful to the Lord."[42] One can only wonder how that statement affected the panicky families of the twenty-six children who were not dropped off early and who were still missing at that time.

And there is a second cost to some kinds of meaning-making. If a yellow billiard ball rolls into a blue ball, which then knocks a red one into a pocket, you cannot really hold the blue one responsible. After all, it could not control the fact that it was struck by the yellow ball and that that is why it hit the red ball. It was not a "perpetrator" really, more a "victim." Earlier, in Chapter 4, I discussed the long history in psychology of not holding sex offenders responsible for their behavior. The behavior was, it seems, the fault of their "frigid" wives or "seductive" child victims. It was a symptom of family dysfunction. We mute the realization of malevolence—which is too threatening to bear—by turning offenders into victims themselves and by describing their behavior as the result of forces beyond their control.

Dr. Lerner described this process of shifting and denying responsibility well:

> Consider the following set of circumstances. I am assigned responsibility at the clinic for a patient who is a "sex offender." During the initial sessions I spend hours listening to the details of the patient's perverted assaults on young girls and boys, while probing for some understanding of the meaning of these acts in terms of their patient's past history—what had been done to him. . . . And although I may not find this sex offender particularly admirable, it is virtually inevitable that I will view him as the "innocent victim" of circumstances that were inflicted upon him by his genes and the events that happened to him, especially as a youngster. There will be little if any tendency to condemn him for the evil acts he committed: after all, given the chain of events involved, I realize that *he* was not the "real cause"; he was just the transmitter of a series of antecedent conditions.[43]

There are no perpetrators in this nifty—and just—world we construct, and no innocent victims either, not really. What seems like a perpetrator is actually just another victim, and what seems like the victim of his brutality is really someone who shouldn't have gone out at night in the first place and thus is responsible for not avoiding the assault. Easy to bring the world quite round if you work at it.

Oddly then, in our search to find meaning, we often assign victims too much blame for their assaults and offenders too little. Our inconsistencies do not seem to trouble us, but they are truly puzzling. After all, if the offender is not to blame for his behavior, why would the victim be, no matter what she did or didn't do? Our views make sense, however, if you think that we are trying to reassure ourselves that we are not helpless and, that, in any case, no one is out to get us.

Impact of Positive Illusions on
Mental and Physical Health

Positive illusions may cost us in some ways—in our treatment of victims, in our contact with predators—but there is also little doubt that these same illusions cause people to be happier and healthier and to function better. This is important because it suggests the answer is not going to be simply to give them up (even if we could).

Studies on health, for example, suggest that those with positive illusions stay healthier and tolerate serious illnesses better than their more realistic counterparts. Research on AIDS, for instance, suggests those who hold unrealistically positive views about the course of their illness are more likely to live longer and to have a slower onset of the illness than those who don't.[44] In addition, results of a study by Dr. Shelly Taylor indicated that self-enhancement—having an inflated opinion of oneself—was positively correlated with good relations with others, personal growth, purpose in life, self-esteem, mastery, and self-acceptance.[45] It was negatively correlated with state anxiety, depression, self-blame, and neuroticism. In short, those who held positive illusions about themselves scored better on standardized tests of mental health than their more negative peers.

There are critics on the subject of positive illusions, of course, but even they have mostly admitted that such illusions exist and appear to be widespread.[46] The argument seems to focus more on the mental health of those who hold them. Such critics charge that self-enhancers are narcissistic[47] and poorly adjusted.[48] In short, critics claim, self-enhancers may exaggerate their degree of healthy functioning just as they exaggerate everything else.[49] The idea that they are healthier than others is just another positive illusion.

But that dog won't hunt. Dr. Taylor and colleagues, for example, found that there was no correlation between indicators of illusory mental health and self-enhancement. In addition, the findings in this study didn't change when mental health was assessed by self-report, trained peer judges, or friends. In short, there was no evidence at all that "self-enhancers" were less well-adjusted than other people and a good deal of evidence to the contrary.

The most intriguing part of the study, however, was the finding that on physiological measures of stress, self-enhancers showed *more* resistance to stress than did low self-enhancers, not less, as they should if they were really hiding their distress. They not only had a healthier physiological response to stress deliberately induced during the experiment but also lower baseline cortisol levels, which suggests that self-enhancement may have protected them from stressors in the past.

In short, it really does look like people who are optimistic, hold positive illusions about themselves, and "self-enhance," are healthier physically and emotionally than those who don't. No wonder Lionel Tiger wrote that, "Private optimism is a public resource. Public optimism is a private facility."[50] If the world held no predators—or if they were far rarer than they are—this would be a done deal: Take any positive illusion you can find and run with it.

My argument is simply this: Most people think offenders take advantage of our vulnerabilities, and they do. If a child molester can find a lonely child or an overwhelmed single mom worried about her son having a male role model, he will sidle in like a viper slipping into a nest with baby birds. But the genius of predatory behavior is not just that it feeds parasitically on our vulnerabilities, but that it turns our strengths against us as well.

Normal, healthy people distort reality to create a kinder, gentler world than actually exists. Such distortions work in our favor most of the time and make people happier, healthier, and more effective. Hope is a gift, and if it has a dark side—the lottery has been called a tax on the poor—on sum it likely gives more than it takes. Life would surely provide a hard row to hoe without it.

But violent and sexual predation are not small problems, and they extract a fearful toll. Our assumptions that we can recognize a predator, that people are basically good, that anyone who is likeable is trustworthy, are exactly the illusions that made it little challenge for Ted Bundy to fake a health emergency and to get a young woman to help him to his motel room. Why, that nice young man was obviously in distress. What could happen? It was the middle of the day in a motel corridor with her family right down the hall, no more than a shout away. And that assumes she was even suspicious enough to think about the possibility that something *could* happen.

Afterward, of course—if the victim survives—life looks different. The positive illusions that sustain us can shatter in the face of trauma. And what is left is a very different view of the world.

The Impact of Trauma

It is easier to hold positive illusions if our lives are going reasonably well—by which I mean nothing dreadful is happening. Even serious stressors do not ordinarily shake our worldview, our sense of safety or our positive illusions. We find meaning one way or another. We decide that we could have done something differently. It didn't have to happen. It won't again.

Certainly other people's traumas rarely devastate us, despite the fact we are now instantaneously exposed to every war, famine, earthquake, shark attack, and serial killer around the world. Nonetheless, despite the daily influx of bad news, we maintain our personal sense of invulnerability and safety. Something in us believes that all those terrible things will happen over there, to someone else, but not to us. A logical appraisal of our chances of being victimized may occur in our head but will not reach the heart.

In short, a child who is safe enough, loved enough, and protected enough grows up to be an adult with positive illusions, one who expects to be safe, despite what he or she sees all around. A perfect childhood isn't needed, just an absence of overwhelming trauma.

But what happens when the adult is then exposed to a very serious traumatic event, when he or she is abducted and tortured, when there is a horrific accident, or when a child dies? What happens if he or she winds up in a concentration camp, becomes a paraplegic, or is violently assaulted? People are not always able to come up with a meaning that satisfies. The world does not always seem just, and optimism is not always sustained. In fact, worldview can shift dramatically, and positive illusions shatter upon exposure to severe, personal trauma.

My first exposure to the entire issue of positive illusions came when I saw what severe trauma did to normal people and how they felt about the world. I didn't know there was such a thing as positive illusions until I saw a child without them. It began, for me, with a child I will call Jonathan.

Jonathan didn't seem destined to a traumatic childhood. He was born in a small town in Vermont to a couple who loved each other dearly and who had many strengths and no debilitating problems. In fact, both parents were unusually bright and thoughtful people, and both were exceptional parents.

But his childhood veered suddenly after he and his younger sister began attending a local home day care run by a woman with an adolescent son who sexually abused the children. Eventually, Jonathan disclosed sexual abuse, and although his parents believed him, the other parents did not. They had trusted the day care provider, and their trust wasn't easily shaken. Initially, the other parents raised $1,500 for the legal defense of the day care owner.

That changed when their children too began disclosing sexual abuse. When the dust settled, the adolescent confessed and implicated his uncle who, he said, abused him and joined him in abusing the children. Jonathan had not only been sexually abused by both offenders but had been forced to watch his younger sister be abused and to abuse her himself while the men watched. The evidence was solid on all of this, and both men were convicted in a court of law.

The disclosures explained some things. Jonathan had become very spacey in the time he attended the day care. Even in the therapeutic day care he later went to, he would be found at times wandering aimlessly, most often in the bathroom, not sure of where he was and seemingly without a reason for being there. Also, he had begun to have "accidents." He fell off a roof, shot himself with his father's bee sting kit, and exploded a paint can.

I worked with Jonathan for a couple of years in therapy, and at the end of it he was better. He no longer curled up in a fetal position when he was angry or upset. He had stopped engaging in such risky behavior. He no longer dissociated quite so obviously, and the days of wandering around the school were over.

Still, I did not think him a well child. For one thing, he read—not like other kids, but compulsively and in a way that protected him from social interactions. He read at recess, for instance, instead of playing. But, if you have to pick a way to dissociate, reading beat wandering around the bathroom. He was learning and doing well in school: His head was getting clearer even if his heart was still hunched over.

Then one day when Jonathan was ten years old, he and his parents went to Boston with another family to see a play. They emerged from the theater in mid-afternoon, the street temporarily flooded with theater goers. There were four adults and three children walking on the crowded street, the children walking a few feet ahead of the adults. It was not a dangerous area, nor was it even night. Understandably, no one was thinking about safety.

What happened next happened so quickly that, except for luck, Jonathan's father would have missed it. The father was talking to another adult when he happened to notice a man in the crowd walking toward them with his eyes fixed on Jonathan. His focus was so intent that it seemed odd to the father, and he kept an eye on the approaching man, puzzled but not yet alarmed. Just as the man reached Jonathan, he put his hand on the boy's shoulder and bent down as though to speak to him. Suddenly, he grabbed Jonathan by the arm and started to disappear in the crowd.

Jonathan's father leaped forward when he saw the man's hand move toward his son, and he got his arm around Jonathan's waist as he was disappearing in the crowd. The man let go and kept going.

The next morning Jonathan's father sat in my office while Jonathan waited for his turn. His father's face was gray, and he looked ill. "It was so fast," he said repeatedly. "You wouldn't believe how fast it was. The whole thing was just a few seconds. No one saw it. None of the other adults saw it. It was just so fast." And then he added, "I don't know why I'm so upset. After all, nothing happened."

I had a feeling a whole lot had just happened. But I was wrong. A whole lot had happened a long time ago, and I had missed it.

When Jonathan came in, he sat down calmly. "I don't know why my father's so upset," he said, "bad things are always going to happen to me."

"Huh?" I said.

"Well, they will," he went on. "I've always known that," and he took some paper and drew a child standing under a cloud, rain pouring from the cloud merging into tears from the child's eyes.

I had known in the time I had treated this child that he was ashamed and guilty over molesting his sister, that he was frightened of the offenders, and that he dissociated to get away from the whole mess. But what I hadn't known was that his entire view of the world had changed. He had gone from expecting good things of the world to feeling, as he said, that there was no such thing as good luck, only bad. Far from feeling safe and invulnerable, he didn't expect to live to adulthood. "What would have happened if the guy had snatched you?" I asked him.

"Oh, he would have killed me," he said matter of factly. Not a surprise to him. If it wasn't this guy, he added, it would be someone else.

My client had developed what I now call a trauma-based worldview. It was little known in the field of sexual abuse at the time, but I found pockets of research on it in the larger field of psychology, mostly under the term "shattered assumptions."[51] In fact, researchers had been documenting for well over a decade what trauma does to the positive illusions that cushion and sustain us. Severe trauma fosters a very different worldview, one in which the world is no longer meaningful, in which a benevolent deity does not hover, in which individuals are helpless, and in which safety is a fragile and sometime thing. The world seems random at best, malevolent at worse. And children are as susceptible as adults.

On July 15, 1976, in Chowchilla, California, a school bus ambled along a country road, dropping kids off from summer school.[52] A broken-down white van appeared ahead, partially blocking the road, and the bus driver slowed to pass it. To say he was not concerned is an understatement. It was a normal summer day in a small town in the United

States during the 1970s. The driver was making a routine trip along a familiar route with his regular group of school kids, wet and tired from a swimming trip. There was no ominous sound track to alert the driver that he and the children were in harm's way.

All of that changed when he slowed the bus and a man with a mask and a gun jumped out of the van and ordered the driver to open up. Another man appeared with a stocking over his face. Both got on the bus, and one took over the driving while an accomplice followed in the white van.

The kidnappers drove the bus into a ravine and loaded the children and the driver into two vans, the white one and a second green one. It was pitch black in the back of the vans. There was no water, no food, no place to go to the bathroom, and it was very hot in the California summer. It was also hard to breathe in the closed truck. The kidnappers started driving, and the children bounced and jostled on the wooden seats, getting hungrier and thirstier, sweating endlessly and eventually urinating on themselves—for the next eleven hours. The vans stopped some time around 3:00 A.M.

When the vans finally did stop, the children were taken out, and a kidnapper questioned each child in turn, asked their full name, and took an object from each of them, presumably to prove identity. The questioning must have frightened the children terribly. They were each brought in one by one and confronted by strange men with guns. After questioning, each child was forced to climb down a ladder into what appeared to be a hole in the ground.

What looked like a hole from above turned out to be the entrance to a truck buried below. The interior was lit with flashlights. There were some stale snacks left out and cans of murky water. No doubt, it seemed better than being squeezed together in the pitch black vans— that is, until the children heard the sound of shoveling.

Panic set in at this point. They were being buried alive. The bus driver, Ed Ray, begged the men for mercy, but no one answered. Eventually the shoveling stopped, and the men went away. Hours dragged by. The flashlights began to burn out. The children cried and prayed and finally sat numbly. Some slept.

There were twenty-seven people in a twenty-five-by-eight foot truck. The air was hot and muggy and breathing was difficult, as it had been in the boarded up vans. There were two fans set in ventilator shafts, and it was obvious to the bus driver they were being run by batteries. When those batteries died, he realized, so would they. There was nothing to do but try to get out.

It wasn't easy. A heavy steel plate had been put on the entrance to the hole and two one hundred–pound batteries on top of that. There were boards nailed together beyond that and dirt on top of the boards. It took hours and phenomenal effort to move the steel plate aside, remove the batteries, and complete the tedious work of prying the boards apart and scooping out the dirt on top, handful by handful. The bus driver and two of the older kids, fourteen-year-old Mike Marshall and eleven-year-old Roberto Gonzales, led the effort.

They had no tools—they took a mattress apart to get coils to pry up the boards. They had no room, and they were working over their heads. They were exhausted and frightened and slowly suffocating. Still, they persisted. They took turns digging. Some watched the younger children while others worked. One held a flashlight. Another removed the dirt below.

After sixteen hours in the buried truck, Mike Marshall climbed out of the truck, sure the men with guns would shoot his head off. He called down to say no one was there, and one by one the bus driver handed out the other children. No one had a clue where they were. They saw a light in the distance and went toward it, still fearful it could be the kidnappers. But instead they found two workers at a rock quarry who instantly realized who they were. One called the police, and almost within minutes a blinding array of lights and sirens descended on the bewildered children. The police tried to load the children on buses to take them to the hospital for evaluation, but it proved difficult. The younger kids kept slipping off and hiding. They had no faith in buses.[53]

The behavior of the kids was a clue to what was little understood in 1976, that trauma that did not leave physical scars could leave emotional ones that would prove longer lasting and harder to heal. At the time, the physicians who examined the children pronounced them well. The town, understandably, rejoiced at their return "unharmed" and put a brass plague on a boulder to thank God that nothing bad happened. Better to thank God that nothing *worse* had happened. Because something very bad had, indeed, happened, and the children did not come back the same children that left the day before.

Lenore Terr is a tenacious trauma researcher who saw in Chowchilla the case study for which she was looking. She called the parents after the children's return and arranged to evaluate all the kidnapped children as well as a little boy who was one of the children let off the bus before the white van stopped it. Four years later she evaluated them again.[54] She also studied control samples, children in other similar towns who had not been part of any known traumatic event to date.

It is not clear how much the children liked Lenore Terr: One child joked five years later that his only lingering fear was of psychiatrists.[55] It is also not clear how much she helped them in the brief time she worked with them, but that was not her purpose. She saw herself as a scientist conducting a crucial research study, and unlike almost anybody in the late 1970s, she knew what she was seeing. What she documented in dry scientific language and meticulous detail was what being kidnapped and buried alive on a sunny day on your way home from summer school will do to a bunch of normal kids. What it did was to produce "massive interferences with optimism and trust."[56]

After the kidnapping, many of the Chowchilla children were no longer friendly or open or trusting. Sunny children with gentle dispositions turned sullen, even rageful, and their sense of the world changed as much as their temperaments. It was no longer a safe and benign world. Like Jonathan, they no longer assumed they'd live to adulthood. One child, nine years old at the time of the kidnapping, decided the Russians were ruining the ozone layer and that everyone would be killed. Another, ten years old, believed the world would end in the year 2000, although his family did not share his views. He wanted to live alone in the mountains when he grew up: Cities and towns were not safe. Twenty-three of the twenty-five children were afraid of the future.

To protect themselves, many children decided they were clairvoyant, and they began to believe in signs and omens. In retrospect, they were sure they knew something was going to happen the day of the kidnapping, and they continued (after the fact) to believe they could predict events. For example, when one child's stepfather died several years later, the child decided he had predicted it in advance, although he had said nothing to his family.

In short, the children no longer felt invulnerable; they no longer believed they were safe; in fact, they no longer felt like they had any power at all. They had developed a trauma-based worldview. And these were the children that everyone thought had emerged unharmed. Instead, Terr found every child had been affected, every single one, for at least the five years she studied them. The occasional contacts she had years later told her that time did little to soften the impact.

It was also striking how similar the Chowchilla children were to other children she treated who had been sexually or physically abused. She quoted one such patient as saying:

> When you get old, you die. I have grandparents who are sixty or sixty-nine and I don't think *they* are ready to die. But I sometimes think I am going to die sooner than other people—I don't know why I think this. I think bad people will hurt me. I may be killed instead of dying.[57]

The child who said this was not a Chowchilla child but rather a little girl who, like Jonathan, had been sexually abused in a day care center. But the abuse had been much younger—from ages fifteen to eighteen months. It happened when she was so young that she could not report the abuse, nor did she appear to even remember it when she was brought in to see Terr at age five. Still, the abuse was certain—it was discovered when pornographic photos of the child came to light, taken by the offenders while they were in the act of abusing her and the other children.

For the child, all that was left consciously by age five was a bad feeling about the day care but no specific memories. Nonetheless, neither young age nor her lack of memory helped her escape the impact of trauma. And once again, it was her sense of safety and her belief in what the future held for her that were affected.

Life after trauma is a different animal altogether, and it is not just different emotionally, it is different cognitively. A study by Dr. Richard Famularo found those with chronic posttraumatic stress disorder, a frequent sequelae of trauma, expected life to be short, difficult, and hard.[58] The researcher Ronnie Janoff-Bulman and colleagues have documented systematic changes in the victim's sense of how meaningful, orderly, and predictable the world is.[59] For many trauma victims, the world simply stops making sense. It is no longer a nifty world or a fair one. Vice is not necessarily punished, nor virtue rewarded. The "rumor of angels"[60] turns out just to be a rumor, after all. As Dr. Daniel Spiegel put it, trauma leaves victims with:

> A marginally bearable sense of helplessness, a realization that one's own will and wishes become irrelevant to the course of events, leaving either a view of the self that is damaged, contaminated by the humiliation, pain, and fear that the event imposed; or a fragmented sense of self.[61]

It is disorienting to go to bed one night only to look out the window the next morning to find a different landscape, one you don't recognize. The bewilderment of the person who loses their sense of meaning in the world is profound:

> We tell ourselves stories in order to live. . . . Or at least we do for a while. I am talking here about a time when I began to doubt the premises of all the stories I had ever told myself. . . . I was supposed to have a script, and had mislaid it. I was supposed to hear cues, and no longer did. I was meant to know the plot, but all I knew was what I saw. . . . flash pictures in variable sequence, images with no "meaning," beyond their temporary arrangement, not a movie but a cutting room experience.[62]

Although Joan Didion does not tell us where her own disorientation came from, and I do not know that it was traumatic in origin, still the landscape she described illustrates well the view of many trauma survivors.

We take the meaningfulness and predictability of the world for granted. We think it is "out there," not a construct inside our own heads. It is only when it shifts and shatters that we are left wondering why we ever believed in it in the first place. It is so obvious, we say, that the world isn't fair, that bad things happen. We knew it cognitively all along. Worse, we lose not just the sense of personal invulnerability, but the sense of personal efficacy as well. The mountains, we realize, really don't care. As Didion complains:

> The universe that suckled us is a monster that does not care if we live or die—does not care if it itself grinds to a halt. It is fixed and blind, a robot programmed to kill.[63]

But believing that is a hard way to live. Life becomes a sentence, not a gift. Time on this planet feels like the enemy. It is beyond this book to talk about the road back from such an altered life. I discussed what I know of it previously in a book on the impact of sexual abuse called *Transforming Trauma*.[64] But the purpose of this book is to try to prevent it in the first place.

Although nothing but good luck will make you and me *completely* safe from predators, it is time to sum up what is known of how they operate and how the illusions that sustain us give them an opening. It is time at least to consider how we might reduce our vulnerability without giving up our hopefulness, our good will, and our joy.

10

Detecting Deception

One must have a mind of winter
To regard . . .
Nothing that is not there and the nothing that is.[1]

What all of us would like is a checklist that we can use to spot predators, a sort of nontechnical polygraph that would tell us whom to
trust and whom not, something on which we could just check off the
items and add up the points.

Unfortunately, such a checklist does not exist.

Even if it did, I believe we would only apply it to strangers and a subset
of strangers at that: those who are *not* charming and friendly, men who do
not look like the boy next door. Certainly, we would not apply it to our
friends and neighbors, not to the neighborhood soccer coach or (until recently) the priest in the local parish that we have known all our lives. We
would not apply it to these people because over and over we confuse likability with trustworthiness, familiarity with safety, warmth with caring.
"Niceness is a decision," Gavin De Becker wrote, but we really don't believe that. Predators, we think, should at least have the decency to be rude.

Before we can deal with any commonsense precautions we could take to
make ourselves and our children safer, we must deal with the tension between the kind of world we want to live in and the kind of world we actually
inhabit. We must deal with the fact that what are called "positive illusions"
give us joy, which can leave us unprepared. But surely the answer is not ter-
minal pessimism, suspiciousness, and fear. What would we be saving then?

The researcher Dr. Ronnie Janoff-Bulman considered these issues
thoughtfully and wrote:

The key to the good life might well be illusions at our deepest, most generalized level of assumptions and accuracy at the most specific, least abstract levels.[2]

In short, there may be little harm in holding generalized expectations that the world will treat us well—so long as we prepare for a world that may not. What is wrong with believing you can learn to swim if you want to? The problem comes if you think you can swim without learning how. Likewise, few of us go on a car trip expecting a wreck— why would we go? But our expectation of a safe journey does not stop us from fastening our seat belts.

We must monitor our illusions—which means becoming conscious of them—and use them discerningly. There is no harm in believing that the future holds more than the past, or that life is basically good, or that good triumphs over evil—in the afterlife if not always here on earth. Those who hold such general and abstract beliefs about the world are more likely to be happier and healthier than those who don't. Neither do I argue with religion for those who choose it—so long as one distinguishes between religion and the men and women who join religious orders.

But where our illusions become dangerous is when they cause us to assume that specific people and situations are not dangerous, when they allow us to assume the best about others without considering the worst. Just because we don't *think* our local priest, youth minister, or baseball coach is a predator doesn't mean he *couldn't* be. We must act as though the world could be dangerous, even if we believe it will not be.

There is some evidence that people are capable of this kind of flexible use of positive illusions. In fact, Taylor and colleagues have steadfastly maintained that positive illusions are not fixed and rigid but can ebb and flow with the situation. Some research findings have suggested that people are more likely to have positive illusions when they are implementing a decision rather than when they are making one.[3] And why not? The decision-making process may be better served by a more deliberate and balanced mindset, whereas once committed to a course of action, enthusiasm becomes a plus.

Monitoring positive illusions is important because most child molestation—even most rapes—begin not with violence but with deception. Even among sadistic rapists, 80 percent will use conning and manipulation to lure the potential victim to an isolated setting.[4] Although it is hard to do anything when facing a man with a gun—and there are a minority of offenders who simply assault—it is not hard to get away from those who con and manipulate if they are recognized early. But that is the issue: recognizing them amid all the similar situations we face each day that are safe.

Even as I write this, I note in the paper this morning that a serial killer is loose in Baton Rouge. Women are buying guns and standing three-deep at practice ranges to learn how to use them. It is not likely to do them any good at all. In all three cases, the assault began at the victim's home, and in none of them was there any sign of forced entry. This killer simply has the ability to get women to open the door to him. Once he's inside the home, there is no time to get a gun, likely not even time to raise one if you had it in your hand. The important moment is the one when he is outside the door, when you are deciding to open it or not. It needs to cross your mind and mine that the friendly looking man wearing a delivery uniform might not be what he seems. We must recognize and modify our own tendencies to believe that we're living in a safe world, in order to live in a safer world.

What Is There to Detect?

If the first step is recognizing our own biases, the second step is to recognize what it is that we are trying to detect and why it is difficult to do so. What mistakes would a child molester or potential rapist make in the conning phase of offending? For what are we looking?

Consider John, an athletic director at a middle school. John has been at his job for fifteen years. He is a genuinely nice man with a pleasant personality. He is outgoing in a gentle sort of way. People like him when they meet him. He listens to others and is neither overtly narcissistic nor controlling. He is warm but low key.

Certainly, he has an excellent work history and reputation at the school. If he's given an assignment, he makes sure it happens. On his own, he develops a variety of sporting activities for children, and he runs them well. Both his organizational skills and his patience in dealing with kids are well known.

He is also a child molester. When the real John was caught, he estimated he had more than 1,000 victims. Over the years, several children had complained to their parents of molestation, but as documented earlier in this book, the children were told that there must be some mistake. John would never do anything like that. He just wasn't that sort of person. In fact, John had grown so confident of this response over the years that he would rape and molest victims in his office with the door shut and a gym full of people in the next room.

In my world, John would automatically be considered high-risk because of his occupation, his long-standing lack of interest in either adult male or female sex partners, and his exclusive focus on activities with children. But for the moment, let us ignore that and focus on the interpersonal interaction.

You are talking with John while your eight-year-old son looks on. He wants to know if your son can go with him and a group of boys to a ball game. Because the park is some distance away and they are leaving early in the morning, John thought he'd just let the kids sleep over the night before. That way the parents wouldn't have to get up early. Is that OK? John's presentation to you is soft-spoken and slightly diffident, nothing pushy. He seems genuinely to like your child, which you think is entirely understandable because you think your child is pretty terrific too.

Your son is looking at you, practically holding his breath he is so excited at the thought of going. You remember guiltily that you had been planning on taking him to a major league ball game, but you've been so busy lately you haven't gotten around to it. This seems like a great opportunity. And you know very well the other children will be allowed to go. Your son takes your hand and says, "Please, Mom, can I go?" If you say no, you are going to be perceived as the latest reincarnation of Harry Potter's Lord Voldemort.

It is not, by the way, an accident that John will ask you in your son's presence. He does not want you to have time to think about this. He wants you to have to disappoint your son if you say no. He knows his "hit" rate is better if the child is present when he asks.

So you are under considerable pressure to say yes, and in addition, you would like to. You want to believe this to be a safe situation, that a nice man could ask your son to a ball game, and that could be all there is to it. Besides, the other kids will be there, and there's safety in numbers, isn't there? You've known John for years. He's thought well of in the community. It's not like you're letting your child go off with a stranger.

What is there on the other side? What reason do you have to say no? If he is a child molester, for what exactly are you looking?

That is the crucial question that most people rarely ask themselves. Are you looking for lying? If so, what is he lying about? Is he lying about taking your child to the ball park? Certainly not. He'll definitely take him to a ball game. Is he lying about his feelings? Does he really like your child? That depends. He may, and he may not. He may be the sort of predator who is not at all interested in your child except for sex. What follows below is an apology letter written by a pedophile who manipulated a boy with a difficult family situation. The pedophile deliberately became the "parent" this child never had, taking him to ball games, buying him gifts, showering him with attention. His apology letter afterward reveals his true interests.

> I am writing this letter to you to let you know the facts of what I did to you. What I wanted from you was your young body to satisfy my lust. I did not love you. I only gave you toys so you would not tell about what I was doing to you, and to make you think good things of me. . . . You may remember the days out I took you on and said I enjoyed those days. I did not enjoy those days with you. I only wanted to see you so I could abuse you.[5]

This "apology" letter was never sent to the child. Although the letter was accurate, it was also very hurtful. The offender's therapist used it in the process of the offender's therapy but did not impose it on the child.

This type of callous attitude is not uncommon in child molesters. As noted previously, a man who sexually abused his toddler stepdaughter said, "It was sex. That was it. I didn't care about, really honestly, I didn't love the child. I wanted the child for my own purposes."

However, sometimes the degree of callousness chills even those who are familiar with it. I once testified against a priest who had sexually abused a teenage boy (along with a number of other children he molested). One day the priest took the child on a trip to visit a rectory in a nearby town. He took the child to a bedroom and told him to "just do as I say," and that if he didn't, their relationship would be over. He made the child strip and left the room.

A few minutes later a man came in the room and anally raped the child. The child started to sob, and the man told him to be quiet. When he finished, the man left without a word. The child was sobbing and bleeding from the anus when another man came in. He thought this man might help him, but he raped him also. Then the priest came back and simply said, "let's go." He never mentioned what happened, just got the child dressed and took him to dinner and a movie.

If you're wondering about motive in this case, consider that that priest also molested another child while he was in counseling for confirmation and told the child he could earn between $200 and $250 for having sex with men. I have no doubts the two men in the rectory paid the priest to rape the child. No, I do not think this priest cared about the child.

However, John, the athletic director who is waiting for your answer, may or may not be as intentionally predatory as those above. He may be the variety of child molester who "falls in love" with each child and becomes obsessed by them. His expression of liking and interest then would be genuine. Where's the lie?

This is an important point because ordinarily, he will carefully avoid telling you any outright lies. The only thing he could be lying about is his intention, but then you aren't discussing that, are you? If he is "lying," it is primarily a lie of omission. He's not telling you what else he's going to do aside from taking your child to a ball game. But lies of omission are hard to spot and easy to get away with. How do you evaluate something someone didn't say? Everything he said was the truth. He just left a few things out.

You could, of course, ask him if he's a child molester, and then he would be forced to lie. But you have no clear reason to do that, and it would be a disastrous strategy. If you ask every pediatrician, youth worker, friend, acquaintance, teacher, therapist, religious leader, friend, and family member if they are child molesters, you will soon have a personal community very concerned about your mental health. And you would alienate all the people who aren't child molesters.

Of course, John is fooling you, and he knows it. The most you are likely to detect is his attitude toward tricking people. Most people assume someone tricking them or lying to them will feel guilt, and they look for conventional wisdom signs of guilt—lack of eye contact and fidgeting. But let us assume for a moment that John is a very predatory offender, perhaps a psychopath, in which case, he will feel something very different when he is lying: He will feel not guilt but joy. He will feel "duping delight." But few people expect to see joy when someone is lying. And even if they did see joy, how can they tell whether the joy is from deception or because John is excited about going with the kids to a Major League ball game?

Even if John is not a psychopath and has a normal amount of guilt and a conscience, he has long ago medicated it through "thinking errors," beliefs such as "children should be free sexually," "he wants it too," and "it won't do him any harm." If so, he will not show signs of guilt because he won't feel it.

Finally, even if he does feel guilt, he will hide it well. There is a category of liar that is particularly hard to detect, called "practiced liars."[6] After years of practice, normal signs of guilt and anxiety wear off. Remember the offender who said to me, "You don't get this, Anna, do you? . . . I've been lying every day for the last twenty-five years." John has been doing this for a long time, and his confidence is high. He has been through this many times before, and even on those rare occasions when a child disclosed the abuse afterward, nothing ever came of it. So what has he to fear? In his mind, nothing. You will see no signs of nervousness or fear from a man who has succeeded in fooling others for more than fifteen years.

What is it you would see, then? What is there to detect?

Very little. For this reason, I do not recommend detection as the main method of protecting our children from child molesters. In Chapter 11, I will talk about deflection, a more effective method than detection. However, even though I don't believe every lie can be detected or every sex offender spotted, I do believe we could do a much better job than we do now. This chapter will summarize what we know about detecting lies in people like John.

Detection

Most liars are not caught because someone spotted a lie in an interpersonal interaction. The most common way that lies are detected is that liars either contradict themselves at different times, or they say things that listeners find out through outside sources are not true. An astonishing number of times, that information is simply ignored or overlooked if the liar is personable enough and glib enough. Even when questioned, a good liar can explain almost any discrepancy. Needless to say, it is a premise of this book that contradictions and discrepancies should be valued more than opinions based on charm or personality.

Nonetheless, there is a large literature on detecting deception through personal interaction alone, and it is useful to know something about it. The most important points are that: 1) people aren't very good at it; 2) people think that they are; 3) the things most people believe will detect deception actually won't; and 4) the things that will detect deception are subtle, easy to miss, and not well known.

Because the first two points have been covered previously, I will restrict this section to the latter two. In an interpersonal interaction, there are only a few major channels of communication that are being used: 1)words; 2) voice characteristics (pitch, rhythm); 3) facial expressions; and 4) body language. Let's start with what won't work and move on to what will.

What Won't Work: Gaze Aversion and Fidgeting

Conventional wisdom tells us that eye contact is a sign of truthfulness and gaze avoidance a sign of lying. But it is not so. It has simply not been found in the research on lying as a sign of deception. Gaze aversion does occur, of course, and may accompany certain emotions—that is, if the person feeling them doesn't deliberately control the direction of his gaze. Paul Ekman has written:

> The gaze is averted with a number of emotions: downwards with sadness, down or away with shame or guilt; and away with disgust. Yet even the guilty liar probably won't avert his gaze much, since liars know that everyone expects to be able to detect deception in this way. . . . Amazingly, people continue to be misled by liars skillful enough to not avert their gaze.[7]

When I train on detection of deception, I ask audiences how many people have heard that gaze aversion is a sign of deception. Inevitably, every hand in the room goes up, and then I ask, "If everyone here knows this information, who else knows it?" The truth is, every sex offender you will ever meet (including young sex offenders just starting out) knows that gaze aversion is thought to be a sign of lying.

There are only two categories of clues that are reliable in terms of detecting deception: 1) signs that the liar doesn't know to fake; and 2) signs that the liar can't fake. If a "sign" doesn't fit into one of those categories, it will not detect deception. Anything a skillful liar knows he or she *should* fake and that he or she *can* fake, *will* be faked. Gaze avoidance fails on both accounts. Not only does every single liar know it's supposed to be a sign of deception, but everybody can control the direction of his or her gaze.

Gaze avoidance, in any case, is not a sign of lying per se but rather is a sign of nervousness, embarrassment, sadness, disgust, or guilt in people who are not practiced in deception. Ironically, these feelings occur more in victims who are telling the truth than they do in sex offenders who are lying.

Acts of touching, rubbing, picking at, scratching, or somehow playing with some part of one's own body are called "manipulators." Outside the technical literature, they are more often simply called "fidgeting." Manipulators can be a sign of nervousness in people who are not practiced in deception. They are not necessarily a sign of deception, however, because many liars, particularly psychopathic ones, do not feel nervous when they lie, and others who are not psychopathic but are practiced liars have had enough experience that they can successfully hide their nervousness.

Thus, using manipulators to assess deception is problematic. They are a sign of being nervous, not of lying. Innocent people, afraid of not being believed, are sometimes more stressed out than guilty people who feel "duping delight" when they pull one over on others. And even those liars who don't feel duping delight and are initially nervous about detection will have lost their nervousness long ago. Don't expect these latter offenders to show manipulators any more than you expect a good actor to do so when he walks on stage.

Consequences and Confidence

All liars, whether they feel guilty or not, respond in some way to a consideration of the stakes and are also affected by their confidence level. High stakes and a target known to be good at detecting deception increases "detection apprehension" or fear of getting caught. Low stakes and a gullible target decrease it. The fear of being detected will work as effectively as guilt in producing nervousness and mistakes in liars. Conversely, the lower the fear of detection, the more chance even an unskilled liar will have the confidence needed to succeed.

We do not ordinarily think this way. Parents generally consider that guilt over abusing a child or betraying a trust would be a major factor for a coach, music teacher, therapist, family member, or friend who is secretly abusing a child. But generally, it is not. Guilt is not a wild thing. It is not a wolf that patrols its territory, forever suspicious and alert. It is more like the family dog who barks at the strange but not the familiar and can be trained in any case.

Guilt can be medicated either by exposure or by thinking errors. As noted, even sex offenders with a conscience will develop a variety of thinking errors that will keep their conscience docile. "There's nothing wrong with it," they will tell themselves. "We just live in a repressive society."

Familiarity, too, will likewise decrease guilt and nervousness. The offender below was considered a pillar of the community. He carefully nurtured an image of himself inside and outside his home as an ideal husband, worker, and community member. Because his offending (ninety victims in all) occurred outside the home, even his wife had no idea what he was doing. Initially, the deception bothered him.

To begin with, how I felt about fooling people is what's really hard to describe. I felt ashamed. For lack of a better word to describe it. Because I knew these people were trusting me. . . . When I would lie to them, to start with I felt a lot of shame. But eventually, I had lied so much to, the shame element was no longer there. It was just a matter of keeping my tail covered. Keeping everything covered up.

Other offenders describe a variable response. The youth minister with close to one hundred victims tells us:

At times there was a great amount of shame for being deceitful. At times there was a great amount of pride: Well, I pulled this one off again. You're a good one. You're very capable of doing this. It works for you. There were times when little old ladies would pat me on the back and say, "You're one of the best young men that I ever have known." I would think back and think, "If you really knew me, you wouldn't say that." And it varied.

In any case, the response that conventional wisdom tells us to expect—shame, guilt, nervousness—will not necessarily be there.

But if guilt and shame are not universal factors that accompany lying, detection apprehension is always a factor. All offenders are aware they could be caught and that—in the case of child molestation—the consequences could be dire. Their fear of detection, however, will be different with different people in different settings. If the targets of the lies are thought to be suspicious and skilled at detecting lies, detection apprehension will increase. Conversely, if they are thought to be trusting and gullible—particularly if they are thought to be religious people who look for the good in everyone—detection apprehension will decrease.

When detection apprehension is high, confidence is low, and liars may make mistakes. Conversely, even an unskilled liar will make few mistakes if he or she is totally confident and has little fear of detection. This is one reason you should be active in your children's extracurricular activities: It sends a message that you are an alert parent, and that will increase an offender's fear of getting caught, which, in turn, will increase the chances he *will* get caught.

Ironically, it is possible for detection apprehension to get so low that liars become grandiose and careless and make mistakes that can undo them. An offender may molest a child in a room with the door open and the other parent in the next room. He may molest a child with other children present who are witnesses and can confirm the child's testimony. He may meet friends who have moved far away in a motel halfway between their two towns, play cards in one room, and take breaks to "check" on the kids sleeping in the next room, but instead molest them with the door open but out of sight. He may take a break from watching a ball game at a friend's house to go to the bathroom but walk, instead, into a child's room to molest her.

All these are real cases of offenders who have been caught because their detection apprehension was too low. Every once in a while a parent walks in on one of the above scenes and cannot be convinced they didn't see what they saw. But the sad fact is that for detection apprehension to be that low, the offender has to be successful at molesting children for many years.

Deception apprehension is not only affected by the suspiciousness and skill of the target but by the stakes as well. You would think that the stakes would be universally considered high in child molestation cases, but it is not so. Any offender knows all too well that a child's disclosure matters little if the child is not believed. In interviewing offenders, I have routinely heard them disclose more victims than those for whom they were caught, but that has never surprised me. Other research has convinced me offenders are almost never caught for *all* the molestations and rapes they commit.[8]

What has surprised me, however, is how many times offenders report that children have disclosed the assaults but were not believed. Over time, an offender who has had several children disclose without suffering any consequences loses his fear of getting caught. And he is right. He knows from experience his word will be taken over that of a child.

Likewise, an offender may discover there are minimal consequences to getting caught for reasons entirely unrelated to whether the child is believed or not. The priests making headlines recently as serial predators were sent from parish to parish when their molestations were discovered. They were very likely more believable each time, their fear of being caught lowered, and their confidence increased by their previous experience.

And far from being less likely to continue molesting, they were surely more likely to continue. After the first time, they had to know for a fact that they would be protected if caught, able to maintain their careers and merely given a fresh start, a new parish and a new group of children. Given that, the fact that they continued to molest is hardly surprising.

What all this means is that John, the athletic director asking you to allow your son to spend the night at his house, may have experiences in his background that you can't possibly know about that have made him confident—confident enough that his lies to you will be very difficult to detect even if you are suspicious and knowledgeable. He may have been caught before, but the child was not believed. He may have been caught before but allowed to resign and even given a positive job recommendation. He may have been caught before, but the parent agreed not to report it to the police if he would "just get help."

All of these scenarios are common in the histories of child molesters. All of them make offenders more confident and less afraid of getting caught. John could be a natural liar or a psychopath, but even if he is neither, he is for sure a practiced liar. If he has been caught and let off the hook previously, he is also a relaxed and confident liar. It will take more than bad advice about gaze aversion and fidgeting to catch him.

Bad Liars and Good Liars

It is not only the amount of detection apprehension or an offender's confidence level that determines whether a liar will be detected. There are people who are just plain good at lying and others who aren't worth a damn. The best sort of liar to run into is someone who is just naturally bad at lying. Probably, they'd get a bit better if they kept trying, but I doubt many do. They're caught so regularly early on that it isn't rewarding, and they quit. When asked to lie in experiments, they are so afraid of getting caught that they make mistakes that do, in fact, catch them.

Conversely, research demonstrates that there are also natural liars.[9] The ones identified in a study by Ekman did not differ on personality tests from the rest of the group. They did not appear to lie more often, nor were they less moral or more comfortable with betraying trust. They did not use their gift for lying in irresponsible ways. But they all knew that if they chose to lie, they could get away with it. They had known that from childhood. When asked to lie in research studies, they were simply not detectable.

Most people, however, fall somewhere in the middle. They're neither "born to lie" nor "born to get caught." How good they are at lying depends on how much practice they've had. The average person tells small social lies every day, but few of us live a double life. Our opportunity and experience at high-stakes lying—the sort where you're lying about something that could put you in jail—is pretty limited. Very few of us have ever been suspected of a crime, and fewer still have been interviewed by the police about one. Under such circumstances, detection apprehension would be very high for most of us.

But that would change had we practiced lying over serious matters every day, had we lived a double life, had we been questioned by upset parents or by police numerous times in the past. You are never going to run into a child molester who is not a practiced liar, even if he is not a natural one.

The final group are psychopathic liars. Truly, they are a different animal altogether. A psychopath will positively enjoy lying and go out of his way to lie when there is little or nothing to gain and much to lose. It is an odd business that what the rest of us experience as detection apprehension strikes him as a thrill. He will lie for the sheer joy of it, and he will fool you for the simple pleasure of saying, "Damn, I'm good."

Characteristics of the Target

Characteristics of the target also play a role in whether a lie will be detected. As noted previously, although a very few people are good at detecting lying, in fact the vast majority of us are worse than we think.

However, there is a second characteristic that merits discussion. People are easier to fool if they have a stake in believing the liar. Therapists, for example, who believe that they have successfully treated an offender will be loath to believe that he has gone astray. To face that means that their treatment was a failure and their judgment of the offender flawed. This is true of all of us. We are all biased toward believing what we want to be true.

Recently I was consulted on a case of a sex offender just released from prison and living in a half-way house. In the short time he had been out, he had successfully convinced a parole officer that he was low-risk. He had, in fact, developed a warm relationship with the officer. There was a retarded man also living in the half-way house, and after the offender had been there several months, the retarded man revealed that the offender had been coercing him into having sex. Unfortunately, it was a very credible charge. This offender had a record of molesting vulnerable people, and this offense was similar to previous offenses, although the victim could not have known that.

Nonetheless, when the victim was being interviewed, the parole officer swung into the room and shouted at him, "You're lying. You're lying. If you keep saying things like that you're going back to jail." He refused to believe the victim or even to listen to him. The irony is that this parole officer had a reputation for being tough on offenders. No doubt that was part of it. He could not believe he could possibly have been wrong about this offender. He refused even to consider it or to listen to the evidence.

The officer was pulled off the case because of his obvious bias but went on, nonetheless, to try to help the defense in the revocation hearing. When the offender went on to assault yet another retarded person, the fact that he was still molesting became glaringly clear.

One time I was stopped at a conference by a federal marshal. His job was to set up sting operations for offenders who bought and traded child pornography over the Internet. He told me that whenever they caught an offender with child porn who was in a therapy group, they notified the therapist. He said about half of them thanked him and took it seriously. The other half simply refused to believe it. They would say something like, "He's doing really well in group. I don't believe he'd do anything like that."

If you think you would not be so irrational, consider how you'd feel if there was a question of whether a friend you cared about, a minister you trusted, or a math tutor you hired was a child molester. What would you prefer to believe? That a child is mistaken, or that a man you liked and trusted—and to whom you gave access to your child—is a child molester? What if the accused was someone to whom you were married, someone who helped create your child and whom you loved? Would it be easy for you to believe this person is a child molester? If it would, then you have a very strange marriage and probably shouldn't be there. Anyone who has a higher opinion of their spouse than they do of a leech is going to find this hard to accept.

What this means is that you have done half the work for the offender. He doesn't have to be all that good if someone is predisposed to believing him. If you have an unconscious bias toward discounting the accusation, you will look for signs that bolster your belief, not for signs that challenge it. Anyone who wants to believe something is easier to persuade than someone who is outside the situation and has no bias either way.

Which brings us back to John. The better you know him, the more you like him, the more stake you have in believing he is not a child molester. You may not have considered the impact your liking him has on your judgment, but rest assured he has. He may not have studied deception, but he has lived it. He has seen firsthand how hard it is for people who like him to believe he's a child molester. So he will work very hard for you to like him. John is a professional operating among kind-hearted amateurs. If you are serious about detecting deception, you must study the very subtle and small signs that will catch John, signs he cannot control or doesn't know to control.

What Will Work: Subtleties and Surprises

I start with considerations of context, confidence, and stakes, and with characteristics of the offender and the target because all of these things affect whether a lie *can* be caught or not. Some lies by certain people in certain situations are simply impossible to detect short of a polygraph.

The polygraph—although not perfect—has a dramatically better track record than mere people in detecting deception.[10] Still, it is mostly infeasible in the myriad of situations you and I face when we seek to determine whether someone could conceivably be a child molester. Assuming the liar is not perfect, assuming you and I are not too biased, assuming there is sufficient detection apprehension and that the liar will make some mistakes, however subtle, what sort of mistakes will he make?

What does detect deception are things to which you and I don't pay attention. When we interact with people, we most often pay attention to what they say and to their dominant facial expressions.[11] We will overlook small irregularities in gesture, pitch, and facial expression in favor of the primary message. Overall, we ask, "Does he look sincere?" "Is he saying the right things?" Even relatively unskilled liars will pass that test.

But the signs of deception in a good liar are subtle and not intuitive. Let's look at these subtle signs of deception one by one and then discuss them in combination.

Emotional Leakage

There is no behavioral sign of deception per se, simply signs of emotional leakage. An offender who is feigning enjoyment of your company may be feeling something very different: fear of getting caught, contempt for how easy people are to fool, anger because he is always angry, even smugness over his own cleverness. Detecting deception really means trying to detect hidden emotion that is at variance with the picture presented to you. Truly, there are no behavioral signs of deception, none at all. Look for emotional leakage.

It follows that almost anyone can get away with a lie that does not involve emotion. If you choose to lie to a friend about something totally inconsequential—how many parking tickets you have—you could almost certainly get away with it. The subject does not involve emotional content. There are no sufficient stakes involved to make you anxious or fearful. Even if caught, you could always say you forgot or that you were embarrassed to admit how many you had, and you would likely be easily forgiven. You know your chances of getting caught, in any case, are small. Your friend would have to find some way to get access to your parking records, and that is unlikely, even if she or he were motivated to try—which is equally unlikely.

However, if you were lying to a friend about having an affair with her husband, the situation would be very different. Your chances of getting caught are greater; the stakes are higher. Also, you probably have feelings about betraying your friend. You would very likely not just be hiding the fact of the affair but would be hiding emotion of some sort as well, whether nervousness, anxiety, fear, guilt, shame, or even triumph, depending on your makeup and your reasons for the affair.

When I began reading the literature on lying and on detection of deception, I looked not just at the psychological literature but at any literature I could find on deception, and I stumbled on the gambling literature. Gambling, of course, frequently involves deception and its detection.

The same principles can be found in the gambling literature that are in the psychological readings. It is as clear to the professional gambler as it is to the psychology researcher that it is emotion, not lying per se, that is detectable.[12] But although high-stakes gambling inevitably involves emotion for the players, it is simply a job to the dealers, and they don't usually get emotional over it.

This latter point is important because it is at times advantageous to be able to read the body language of the dealers, particularly (at one point) in relation to blackjack. At one time dealers often checked their own hole card before offering players the opportunity to take another card. After doing so, the dealer had a pretty good idea whether the player should take the offered card or not, and that knowledge could potentially be read by someone who knew how to read body language. But how to read their body language if emotion wasn't involved and emotion is the only thing that can be detected?

The secret of reading their body language, according to professional gambler and author Steve Forte, is to involve them emotionally in the game. On the surface this would seem like an impossible task. Why should the dealer care? He/she arrives for work day after day, deals a shift, and leaves. Dealers get paid regardless of who wins or loses.

The issue, Forte advises, is to treat the dealer in such a way that he/she ends up rooting for you to win or to lose, which one doesn't matter. To get him rooting for you, compliment him in the presence of the pit boss, tip heavily, ask him for advice, be a good loser, even tip him with your "last" $10 (which should not really be your last $10).

But you could just as easily go the other way. Be obnoxious. Complain about whatever the hotel is most proud of, mumble a lot so she has to ask you to speak up, brag about how good you are, criticize the other players, tip something so small in comparison to your play that it's an insult, take an excessive amount of time to play your hands.

Once the dealer is involved, according to Forte, his or her body language is readable. If she/he wants you to stay, when she offers you a card that she knows you should take, her hand will be in front of her, her body language unconsciously inviting. If she offers you a card that she doesn't think you should take, her hand will be further back or up on her chest, and her body language will be unconsciously discouraging. If you have alienated her, then read her body language the opposite. If she has her hand in front of her, don't take the card; if away, do.

Apparently, Forte's work was so successful that most casinos have changed their procedures since the publication of his book so that the dealer does not know what his/her hole card is at the time they offer other players a card. For our purposes, the point is not whether this currently works, but simply that the more different areas and fields that have found the same principles at work, the more seriously we should take the results.

Gambling takes deception seriously; it's part of the game. And people take gambling seriously because so much money is involved. No doubt gamblers study their field as seriously as psychologists do, although with a different methodology and for a different reason. The principles they have discovered appear to be the same. Emotion is fundamental to the detection of deception.

In conversation, emotional leakage spills out in different ways: facial expression, words, voice characteristics, and body language. We'll look at these channels individually first and then at the issue of harmony and disharmony in the way they fit together.

Facial Expressions

The face and voice are what people generally pay attention to. But these are also the areas that liars pay most attention to. For this reason, those who wish to detect lies might actually be better off focusing elsewhere. Take for example, the following study.

The subjects of the study were nurses, some of whom were asked to watch films of pleasant scenes, others to watch films of gruesome amputations.[13] The nurses were interviewed while watching the films by someone blind to what they were seeing. All the nurses were asked to persuade the interviewer they were watching a pleasant film of flowers as convincingly as possible. The interviews were videotaped.

Later, portions of the interviews were shown to raters who were asked to rate who was lying, that is, who was not watching the pleasant scene even though they said they were. Some raters only saw the facial expressions but did not hear the words or see the body language. Others only heard or read the words. Still others only saw the body language—no face or words. Still others had the voice run through a filter that made the words not comprehensible but left the pitch, rhythm, and so forth intact. In short, Paul Ekman, who conducted the study, managed to isolate the four channels so that each rater only saw one: facial expression, body language, words, or voice characteristics.

Imagine you are rating these films. Which of the four channels of communication—facial expressions, words, voice characteristics, or body language—would you bet on as the most revealing of deception?

If you are like most people, you would say facial expressions or words. But it was not so. The raters who saw the facial expressions or the words did worse in spotting those nurses who were lying. Those who saw the body did best—but best is a relative term. They were right only 65 percent of the time.[14] However, there were clues to deception—not used by the participants—that could be clearly seen on the film by trained observers. Some of the signs that will detect deception but that the raters did not pay attention to are as follows:

Micro Expressions   Emotion hits the face for a microsecond—as little as 1/25 of a second—before the person actually feels the emotion themselves. Obviously, until someone is consciously aware of being angry or afraid, he or she cannot suppress it. When people do register the emotion, they will then squelch the emotion if they do not want an observer to detect it, but a careful observer may spot it anyway in the brief instant that it is on the face.

Squelched Expressions   When the person tries to hide the emotion, you may still see traces of the emotion as they struggle to control it. Obviously, this is a subtle business. The person's face doesn't contort dramatically. Perhaps the eyebrows will lower in anger even as the face displays a phony smile. However, a squelched emotion does last longer than a micro expression even though the end result is usually not a full emotional display, but a section of one, or a blended emotional display.

Automatic Expressions   When people feel emotion, ordinarily those emotions are transmitted to the face without conscious thought. People who are sad look sad and may even cry without making any sort of conscious decision to put a sad look on their faces or to make themselves cry. Of course, the person may try to suppress, control, or hide what they're feeling, but such conscious attempts are necessary because without them the emotions will automatically show.

However, we are actually only dimly aware of what other people see on our faces. Most people's conscious attempts to replicate an emotion they are not feeling often miss subtleties of the contraction of muscle groups that occur freely with unconscious displays. It seems it isn't even the same part of the brain that's involved in conscious and unconscious displays. Individuals with stroke damage to the pyramidal system are unable to smile deliberately, but will do so automatically when they're happy. People with brain damage to the nonpyramidal system show the opposite pattern.[15]

What this comes down to is that certain muscle groups are very hard to control consciously, but they may nonetheless automatically contract during unconscious displays of emotion. For example, when people are sad, their mouths turn down in a frown, and that's what most people remember and try to imitate when they pretend to be sad. It's possible to do so because those muscles are under conscious control.

However, there is another, lesser-known part of a sadness facial display: The inner corners of the eyebrows rise. Most people don't notice this and couldn't control it even if they wanted to. Try raising just the inner corner of the eyebrows alone without raising the full brow. Less than 15 percent of people can do it voluntarily.[16] It turns out the forehead is the most reliable site for determining whether displayed emotions are genuine or not because muscle actions happen there that people cannot easily reproduce voluntarily. In addition to sadness, the eyebrows make a characteristic display for worry, apprehension, and fear: Both eyebrows raise and pull together, a movement that less than 10 percent of people can make voluntarily. (Ordinarily, when people consciously raise their eyebrows, they become further apart.) The eyebrows also play a role in anger and surprise, lowering with anger and rising with surprise, but these actions are also under conscious control and are not reliable indicators.

Smiles   Smiling itself is under conscious control, but there are subtleties that differentiate felt smiles from phony smiles. Felt smiles and phony smiles are different physically: In a felt smile, the entire musculature of the face lifts upward. In a phony smile, only the corners of the mouth lift while the area around the eyes stays smooth and expressionless.

This is the only accurate sign of deception that has begun to find its way into conventional wisdom. If asked, most people will tell you that the difference between a felt smile and a phony smile is in whether the eyes are smiling too. But it isn't clear that most people make use of that knowledge when looking for deception.

In addition, if people are really enjoying themselves, the eyes will light up, regardless of the reason for the smile. Thus, a psychopath who wants to give the impression that he or she likes you may genuinely smile because he is enjoying "duping delight." If so, to all outward appearances, the smile will appear felt—because it is.

A discussion of all the muscle groups that contract with conscious and unconscious displays is beyond the scope of this book. See the writings of Paul Ekman for a more detailed discussion.[17] But the bottom line is that it's often possible to recognize whether an emotion is genuine or not by learning which muscles contract upon involuntary displays and comparing those with the person you are assessing.

Asymmetry   Sometimes an expression is subtly different on one side of the face than on the other. Close scrutiny may suggest that someone is smiling more broadly on one side (a "crooked smile") or that one side shows more anger than the other. This occurs more, it seems, with deliberate, staged displays of emotion than automatic, genuine ones. People don't appear to have perfect conscious control of their faces although they have much better unconscious control of them; in other words, there is less asymmetry when they are actually feeling an emotion. There is some controversy over this finding, but it appears that asymmetry is an indicator that the expression is phony, particularly in the case of smiles.

Timing   Finally, timing—how long an emotion is displayed and when it occurs—may give away the fact that an expression is phony. Felt expressions are displayed very briefly. Any emotion that is displayed for five seconds may well be phony; any expression displayed for ten seconds almost certainly is. Although emotional states last longer than this, the face actually changes expressions. Someone who is angry, for instance, may be angry for a period of time, but his or her face will not hold a single expression of anger during that period. Rather, it will shift to different expressions of anger with different intensities. The shortest emotional expression of all is surprise. Surprise starts, displays, and stops, all within a second. Surprise that occurs longer than that is almost certainly staged.

Timing also refers to when the display occurs. In general, emotional displays that follow words are likely to be false. In genuine emotion, the emotion hits first and then the words follow. Certainly, if a physical display of anger occurs—throwing something, waving a fist—and the angry expression does not precede the display, the anger is likely to be staged.

Body Language

Four aspects of body language have been fairly intensively studied: gaze aversion, fidgeting, illustrators, and emblems. As noted previously, the first two have not fared well in the research despite their general popularity in the world of conventional wisdom. The latter two have fared considerably better.

Illustrators "Illustrators" refer to talking with one's hands. Some individuals and some cultural groups talk with their hands more than others. By itself, talking with one's hands or not doing so means little. Groups and individuals who talk with their hands are no more or less deceptive than groups and individuals who don't. However, research indicates that if someone *does* ordinarily talk with his or her hands, when he/she is being deceptive, he/she does so less than usual.

Why such is the case is not entirely clear, but it's likely for multiple reasons. Illustrators tend to increase when someone is feeling emotional. Thus they may decrease because the person is claiming to be feeling an emotion he or she is not actually feeling. If you're acting happy and excited but you're not feeling it, it may be that your use of illustrators tends to follow what you're really feeling. In addition, it may be that illustrators decrease when people are paying attention to their words, as liars tend to do.

Evaluating illustrators, of course, requires that you know the person's baseline functioning. If you don't know whether the person ordinarily talks with her/his hands, you will not be able to assess whether he or she is doing so more or less than usual. You must first observe the person when he or she is talking about issues that are not sensitive and when you have every reason to expect that the truth is being told. When the topic moves on to areas that are sensitive, note whether the hands become more still or not.

Emblems   The second area where it is thought that deception can be detected is through the leakage of emblems. Emblems are gestures that are self-explanatory within a given culture and do not require words for interpretation. In this culture, they include thumbs up and thumbs down, the peace sign, the hitch-hiking sign, waving good-bye, giving someone "the finger," and more than fifty others. None of these requires a verbal explanation.

If emblems are consciously made—giving someone the finger, for example—they are not signs of deception. Instead, they are nonverbal statements, as eloquent and expressive as words would be. When emblems are signs of deception, they are made unconsciously, and thus they are out of presentation position and often consist of a single element of a gesture rather than the whole gesture. Thus the person's hand may be resting on his hip or leg, with all the fingers pulled back except the middle finger, which may be pointing down. Or the person may push back her glasses with her middle finger.

I mention the middle finger because it is one of the emblems that does leak out. In fact, it was the original impetus for research on this topic. Ekman was doing a study that involved an anger paradigm. In brief, students were being interviewed by one of their (real world) professors about their reasons for going to graduate school. Unknown to the student, the professor was a confederate in the study and had been asked to express contempt for any answer the student gave. If the student stated he wanted to do research, the professor made hostile comments about researchers and then interrupted the student each time he tried to respond. If the student said she wished to do clinical work, the professor made negative comments about clinicians and again interrupted the student rudely each time she responded.[18] The point of the study was to anger the students who would be unlikely to express their anger directly because the professor in front of them was crucial to their success within the graduate school program. In addition, no doubt they were raised to be polite. Under those circumstances, Ekman saw a student quite indirectly give the professor the finger by pointing it down and pulling the other ones back. Ekman knew what he was seeing and quite excitedly commented on it later. To his astonishment, both the student and the professor vehemently denied it had happened. The gesture was unconscious, and thus the student wasn't aware of making it. The professor was sure he would have seen it had it happened. The study was being filmed, and until he showed them the film, neither of them believed him.[19]

What is interesting, of course, is that the emblem was an indirect expression of emotion—in this case, anger. Thus once more, we come back to the notion that it is emotional leakage that is detectable, not lying per se.

The unconscious use of emblems may well be one of the most frequent ways in which emotion leaks when someone is lying. Ekman found that two of the five students in the student/professor anger study leaked emblems, whereas a little more than half of the nurses in the nursing study showed hidden emblems.

The relatively high frequency of hidden emblems may surprise most people because few of us have ever noticed one. However, if you and I don't notice them, it is likely because we aren't looking. The first week after reading the Ekman study above, I was interviewing an inmate with a long track record of child molestation. He was trying to convince me that he was a new man and no longer a threat to children. I had my doubts. In the middle of his attempts to tell me how bad he felt about molesting children, I saw him give me the finger while placing his hand on his hip. What are the chances that nothing like that had ever happened to me before? It seems more likely that I was just never looking for it.

What other emblems could leak emotion? Almost anything. Someone who wants to get rid of you may give an out-of-position wave goodbye. Someone who claims to care deeply about an issue (or a person) may give a one-shouldered shrug or just turn both palms upward. Someone may say "no" while nodding yes or vice versa. Someone who is trying to maintain that he isn't angry may have a clinched fist. Any emblem that expresses an affect in contrast to what the person is saying could be leaking emotions the person is trying to hide.

Voice Characteristics

Voice characteristics refer to everything about the voice except words: pitch, rhythm, stumbling over words, repeating words, and so on. For the average untrained person, aspects of voice characteristics may be more reliable indicators of deception than words are.

For about 70 percent of people, the voice rises when the person is upset. Fear, particularly, appears to result often in raised pitch. Sadness or sorrow tends to result in lowered pitch. In addition, the voice is louder and faster with anger or fear and slower with sadness. These changes appear to be reliable indicators but can be hard to interpret. Is the person afraid because someone has accused them of child molestation, and they are innocent but fearful you won't believe them? Conversely, are they afraid because they are guilty of child molestation and have been found out? If someone gives you the finger covertly, their meaning seems easier to interpret than higher pitch is.

In addition, it is clear that some offenders—psychopaths, for instance—don't experience fear in situations that make other people fearful. "Duping delight" replaces detection apprehension, and duping delight is not likely to cause the pitch to rise.

Repeating words, stumbling over words, and pauses can all be signs that the story line is not flowing naturally and has not been sufficiently rehearsed, in other words, that the person is making it up as he/she goes along. Some liars can be caught this way, but not those who are gifted at lying or psychopathic or even just sufficiently practiced. The voice is a reliable indicator of the emotional state of the person, but it is best to remember that the affective state of some liars may not be what ours would be were we engaged in deception and child molestation.

Still, with all the caveats, in Ekman's study of nurses, a combination of voice measures and facial analysis was able to produce an accuracy rate of 96 percent in detecting deception. In particular, pitch rise and "miserable smiles" (versus genuine smiles) occurred more often in the group of nurses who were seeing a gruesome film of amputations but claiming that they were seeing a pleasant film. In addition, illustrators decreased, and, contrary to conventional wisdom, manipulators decreased as well. However, despite the positive findings on these two body language indicators, it was the combination of voice characteristics and facial expressions that produced the most accurate rates of detection.

I should point out, however, that facial expressions were measured not by simply looking at the faces but by FACS, the Facial Analysis Coding Scheme used by researchers to precisely measure facial expression.[20] The original noncomputerized version of FACS is nothing that ordinary mortals can make use of in the real world. It involves coding forty-four muscle groups in the face for contraction in every frame of film, and it can take up to ten hours to code a single minute of behavior.[21]

When real people saw the interviews, they ignored all of the body language, voice characteristics, and facial expressions that actually detected deception and relied primarily on words alone. Their analysis of words was understandably naïve because they had never been trained in statement analysis, and consequently, they missed the actual clues to deception, focusing instead on signs that did not distinguish the deceptive from the truthful interviews.

Oddly, when people were exposed to only one modality—face, voice, body language, or words by themselves—they tended to focus on the right clues: false smiles, decrease in illustrators, and pitch. But when seeing the full audiovisual presentation, they ignored all of these and focused instead on what conventional wisdom had told them would detect lying, but which would not.

In short, despite the fact that clues were there that could detect deception at a 96 percent accuracy rate, most people were no better than chance in detecting deception. They simply focused on the wrong things. The single exception, as noted previously, was that those who saw the body language alone (with no face or words) had a 65 percent rate of accuracy, better than chance, but which would still have misassigned almost half the subjects.

Words

Words are a little different from facial expressions because they don't automatically pour out when people feel emotion, nor are certain words automatically tied with certain affects. We choose which words we say—more or less. Therefore, a naïve reliance on words will almost always mislead. Remember that the two worst indicators of lying in Ekman's research with nurses were facial expressions and words.

However, just because conventional wisdom hasn't taught us clues to deception in words doesn't mean those clues don't exist. Researchers who study statement analysis think there are clues to deception in words, but not clues an untrained person would recognize. For example, a researcher named Wendell Rudacille has discovered that liars often evade rather than outright deny.[22]

What kinds of evasive answers did people give? What follows is a partial list:

1. Unfinished business: "That's about all." "That's pretty much it"; "That's about all I can remember."
2. Answering the question with a question: "Why would I do something like that?"
3. Maintenance of dignity: "Don't be ridiculous."
4. Commenting on the question: "That's a hard question."
5. Projection: "Someone would have to be sick to do that."
6. Denial of evidence: "You have no proof."
7. Accusation: "Are you accusing me?"
8. Qualifiers: "I can't say"; "I could say"; "I would say."
9. Answers: "My answer is . . . "; "The answer is . . . "[23]

The answers above were intended to reassure the questioner that the person did not commit the crime. But in reality, none of these "answers" addressed the question directly or actually denied the crime. "That's about all," is not the same thing as saying, "That's all." The "about" qualifies the denial. What it really means is "That's not *exactly* all." It is sort of all, mostly all, kind-of/sort-of about all. Which is to say, not all at all.

A different evasion, "I would say," involves a different issue: It's a truism. Ted Bundy could have said, "*I would say* I didn't kill anybody," and it would have been an accurate and true statement. After all, his statement was not that he didn't kill anyone. It was that *he would say* he didn't kill anyone, and that was true.

The basic principle behind statement analysis is that lie catchers should pay attention to what people actually say, not to what they imply. When you read the words literally, you will see marked differences between people lying and people telling the truth. People lying often omit information, evade answering, ask a question instead of answering yours, imply they are innocent but do not actually say it, and the like. It appears that most people don't actually like to flat-out lie. So they find some way to avoid actually lying while satisfying the interviewer's question. This is not to imply that it is a conscious process of evasion, only that empirical observation suggests that's what people do.

Of course, that raises the question as to how often liars and truth-tellers do the opposite: volunteer information that they didn't commit the crime in very specific and nonevasive language. This is termed "spontaneous denial," and it is not denial that is coaxed or forced out of suspects by accusation or pressure. For example, when someone under pressure from press around the world says, "I did not have sex with that young woman," it can be counted as pressured speech, not spontaneous denial. Most people will lie directly if they are pressed hard enough. Accusations, pressure, interrogation, and coercive questioning shape the answers by the refusal to accept evasions. Such tactics often call forth outright denial in someone who would evade the question if left to his or her own devices. To analyze speech, one must have a sample of speech when the person is not being pressured.

Spontaneous denial, then, is denial that pops up in the course of the interview without a great deal of pressure and often even without a specific question on the table. To count, the denial must be very specific and have no evasive elements. Thus, the person must say something like, "I" (first person singular) "did not" (unequivocal) "touch that child's vagina" (specific act), not, "Why would I do anything like that?" or "I would say I didn't do it."

In Rudacille's research, truth-tellers at some point in the interview spontaneously denied the offense 85 percent of the time, whereas liars did so only 7.7 percent. In interpreting all of Rudacille's findings, however, I would caution the reader that although interesting and provocative, there is still only one study on this to my knowledge.

In addition to Rudacille's work, a former member of the Israeli Police named Avinoam Sapir has developed a system of analyzing statements.[24] Sapir is not a researcher and his work is clinical in nature, although, as with Rudacille, there is a single research study to support it.[25] It is a more thorough and comprehensive method of analyzing statements than Rudacille's, however, and if the research continues to support it, this material will be some of the most useful on deception ever developed.

Sapir and Rudacille's methods of analysis are very similar and are the only methods of analyzing offender statements of which I am aware.[26] Sapir agrees with Rudacille that evasive answers are telling. He states in his workshops that, "If he is not committed to the answer, you should not be either." However, he goes beyond Rudacille in developing an entire system of indicators of deception.

Sapir's system analyzes an individual's statement and compares the usual language of the person when he/she is telling the truth with his/her language around the event or issue in question. When people are lying, he finds they differ in subtle ways. Take, for example, the following statement from an interviewee who was a suspect in a homicide investigation. The issue at stake was whether a woman's death by gunshot was accident or murder. Her husband, below, claims that he shot his wife by accident.

Somehow I believe that James [his toddler son] bumped into my right arm and I lost control of the gun. I believe that the barrel was pointing in Nancy's direction and I reacted by grabbing at the gun to get it back under control. When I did this the gun discharged. It went off once and I looked over and saw blood on Nancy's face. I immediately got up and—thinking that I did not want James to see—I think I put something over my wife's upper body.

The point that most of us would pick up on would be how odd the person's response was to the shooting. There is no reference to disbelief or shock or denial. There is no reference to CPR or 911. This makes no sense even if the victim was not his spouse.

And there are other things to be seen even in a single paragraph, some less obvious. In the beginning there are quite a few tentative comments: "*Somehow I believe* that James bumped into my right arm. . . . *I believe* that the barrel was pointing in Nancy's direction. . . ." These are not strong statements, not at all the equivalent of saying, "James bumped into my right arm. . . ." Thus, Sapir would warn us that the husband is "not committed" to the notion that James hit his arm, and if he isn't, then we shouldn't be.

Of course, what is striking is that his lack of commitment comes exactly at the points about which we are concerned. He makes unequivocal statements when describing how the gun went off and killed Nancy—so we know he is not always tentative. But he is wishy-washy when it comes to whether James bumped into his arm and caused that to happen or not, which is precisely the issue that concerns us most.

Finally, what Sapir would point out that few of us would spontaneously consider is that if you look at the husband's description of the whole day, you would find that he referred to his wife seven times. However, in six of those he called her "my wife" and in only one did he call her "Nancy." This occurred only at the time of the shooting.

Sapir's belief is that when people do violence to people to whom they are connected, they distance them in language just as they distance them emotionally. It is even true with guns, he claims. "My gun" becomes "the gun." For arsonists, "my house" becomes "the house" at the time the fire is set.

This is the internal comparison mentioned above, in which a comparison is made between someone's speech at times when they are presumed to be telling the truth versus times when deception is suspected. Such an internal comparison is usually more fruitful than comparing their speech to that of others in that it controls for the natural differences in speech patterns that occur between two people that have nothing to do with deception. If an examination of his speech throughout the day suggested that the husband always called his wife, "Nancy," Sapir might well question how close the relationship was, but he would not think his calling her "Nancy" at the time of the shooting was significant.

Of necessity, this introduction only covers a couple of the principles in Sapir's system of analysis.[27] However, all of the principles are guided by the same notion as is Rudacille's system of statement analysis: We should be paying attention specifically to what people say, not to what they imply or intend to convey. Ordinarily, we help people out by getting the sense of things and filling in the blanks ourselves.

Some of these principles seem obvious in retrospect, but how many of us catch the subtle extensions of them at the time? When Susan Smith, the South Carolina woman who drowned her children by pushing her car into a lake with them in it, went on TV to plead for their "safe return," few of us thought immediately that she likely killed them. An analysis of her language, however, suggested she did. At the time, their father said,

> Everywhere I look, I see their play toys and pictures, . . . They are both wonderful children. I don't know how else to put it. And I can't imagine life without them. [28]

He spoke in the present tense because he knew nothing of the fate of his children and, like all parents who have missing children, he clung to hope.

But while the entire nation felt horribly for the parents and prayed for the safe return of those children, few of us noticed that Susan Smith's language was different. She said in an interview at the same time, "They *were* my life" (italics mine).[29] Note the change in tense. Unlike her husband, she knew they were dead, and her use of language reflected it.

A careful reading of her interviews with police also showed that she exhibited other signs of deception, as when she objected to a police question regarding her knowledge of their deaths by saying,

You son of a b–! How can you think that! I can't believe that you think I did it. . . . I did not have anything to do with the abduction of my children, . . . Whoever did this is a sick and emotionally unstable person.[30]

To a naïve reader, this seems like vehement denial. In Rudacille and Sapir's world, it is not. Indeed, Smith is: 1) objecting to the question; 2) answering a question with a question; 3) saying she "can't believe" he thinks she did it (not that she didn't do it); 4) denying specifically that she had anything to do with *the abduction* of her children (which is true; she killed them but she did not abduct them); and 5) using projection. She used four different evasions in one short statement. "A statement should not whisper deception," Sapir says in his workshops, "It should shout it." In the statement analysis world, Susan Smith shouted it.

Disharmony

More than anything else, it is disharmony that signals deception. When people are telling the truth, their hands, facial expression, voice pitch, and words will be in harmony. When they are not telling the truth, their words may sound truthful but their voice pitch may rise. Or it may be that they have their words and their voice pitch under control, but they may show an emblem, a gesture that is out of synch with what they are saying. They may decrease their use of illustrators or experience a micro expression—a brief, fleeting glimpse of anger may show up just before the smile. One side of the face may have more of an expression of concern on it or more warmth than the other.

But these are small and subtle things. They are not easy to see. They are very easy to miss, and they aren't even always present. Some lies are simply not detectable by anyone. Thus, although I report information on detecting deception, I do so with strong reservations about its effectiveness in protecting our children. We should not put all our eggs into the basket of detecting deception; we should consider deflection instead.

11

Protecting Our Children and Ourselves: Deflecting Sex Offenders

It is hard to remember now, but hospitals were once careless about blood. The gloved and masked creatures our children know as doctors and nurses were once people who actually put their hands on patients without a latex barrier, who smiled without a mask. But then came AIDS, and it became clear that caretakers could not tell who did and who did not have AIDS until after they had drawn blood, after they had exposed themselves to possible infection. And so health care workers simply started treating everyone as though it was *possible* he/she had AIDS. Now they wear gloves with every patient. They use the same blood-handling procedures with everyone, regardless of whether they "look like" they have AIDS or not.

Assume every coach, every priest, every teacher is not *likely* to be a sexual predator, but that one could be and that you will not know if he is. Given that we cannot detect child molesters or rapists with any consistency, we must pay attention to ways of *deflecting* any potential offenders from getting access to us or to our children.

Particularly, we must consider paying attention to probabilities and avoid high-risk situations. For any given situation we must weigh the odds. We must look at someone like John and consider that he works with kids, plays with them after work, focuses his entire life on them. But also consider that the children on whom he focuses the most always seem to be the same age and sex, that he has no adult love interests, and finally that he is seeking an overnight alone with my child. Is there possible risk here? Yes. Can my son go? No.

I do not recommend dropping children off at sports practices and extracurricular activities if you can help it, at least not at young ages. I do not recommend sending them on overnight trips with their coaches or other youth activity leaders without going along. In elementary and middle school, parents can go with their children to the school sock hop, to the community sports practices, to the games. You are not too busy. You can't afford to be.

Just yesterday I took one of my children to his first Little League practice. As I was walking up with my chair and book to watch the practice, a mother called to me from her car. The car wasn't parked but just stopped on the street. "Is this the Little League practice field?" she asked.

"Yes," I replied.

"Is this where Coach Smith's practice is being held?" she asked.

"I don't know," I said. "That's not the name of my son's coach." Still, she did not park. Is she really going to do it, I thought—drop a nine-year-old off for his first practice the first day of the first year of Little League? She isn't sure she's even in the right place; she doesn't know if the coach is here. There are three large practice fields here. How is he even supposed to find out where he belongs? Worse, she is not going to even meet the coach. She's going to send him a message that this kid is on his own. Yes, she was going to do it, and she did.

This afternoon I took my daughter to a soccer practice. There were ten eight-year-old girls, two male coaches, and only two parents there. Eight years old is the average age when sexual abuse starts for girls. Only two parents of these girls would know if there were typical signs of grooming, if girls were being touched unnecessarily and inappropriately, if one or more of them was being singled out for special favors, if one was taken away from the rest of the group for special time. Only two of us.

There is a second gain from being present. A parent who is constantly attending his/her child's extracurricular activities has a less vulnerable child. They do not have a child who is easy to groom because the child is already getting the attention that he or she needs. It is hard to substitute for someone who is there, difficult to worm into a child's affections if she or he has active and involved parents. And it is a signal, too, to pedophiles that you are watching. I do not find that most pedophiles are looking for a challenge; most are looking for an easy target.

Of course, some sports are run by the school, and parents have access to games but not practices. But today, many extracurricular activities in elementary and middle school are community events, and parents can be there even at the practices, cheering their kids on, smiling but quietly watching. Music lessons can take place in your house or in a center rather than the home of the instructor. You can volunteer to be a den mother or father. You can help chaperone an overnight.

You do not have to frighten your children by telling them you are there to make sure they're safe. Tell them you're there because you're interested. I understand you do not believe those coaches, music teachers, and volunteers are child molesters. If you thought that, you would not put your children in their care. But be there anyway because some day one of them could be.

The Catholic priesthood is not the only profession in which pedophilia is an issue. Child molesters have been found in the ranks of teachers, therapists, ministers, Salvation Army staff, police, probation and parole officers, Boy Scout leaders, Big Brother volunteers, camp staff youth workers, priests, doctors, psychologists, and probably every profession that has contact with children. I have an edition of *Sports Illustrated* with a lead article called "Every Parent's Nightmare."[1] The cover is filled with mug shots of child molesters; the caption reads "Who's Coaching Your Kid?". Many of these offenders got to know the child by befriending him or her at a youth activity when the parent wasn't present. The special kind of attention, grooming, and often favoritism they lavish on the child is significantly reduced with a parent nearby or even another adult there to supervise.

Organizations that service youth have begun to grow wiser about deflection. The Boy Scouts now have a policy that no scout leader is to be alone with a child. Scout leaders are to work in pairs, go on overnights in pairs. The Scouts have found through painful experience that they cannot tell—with any kind of screening known to humankind—who will or won't turn out to be a child molester. They know too that letting their thousands of Scout leaders take kids alone on overnights is an invitation to pedophiles to fill out an application.

Whenever possible, it is wise to deflect possible abuse, in other words, be there and supervise your child or support organizations that believe in avoiding situations where sexual abuse is possible. Above all, offenders need opportunities to get to know your child, to gain his or her trust, and finally they need time and a place to abuse them. No opportunity. No abuse.

Playing the Odds

Of course, you can't always be there, and as children grow and achieve more independence, there are more and more situations where you would be thought intrusive and your presence embarrassing to a child. In those cases, you can only play the odds. There are situations where the possibility of molestation is greater or lesser. We can significantly cut down on the problem of abuse by avoiding high-risk situations whenever possible.

Nothing will guarantee that your child won't be victimized in some time and place that you can't stop. I've dealt with confirmed and admitted cases in which a teacher or a principal took kids out of the classroom and molested them in the school. That is not preventable or foreseeable, at least not by the parent, although other teachers may (or may not) have a clue.

But in the majority of cases of child molestation, a parent has been conned into allowing the offender to spend time with the child. In those cases, we have considerably more of a chance to prevent it. One of the ways we can do so is to figure out which situations are high-risk and avoid them. Also, even low-risk situations can be lowered still further with little effort. Other low-risk situations should be avoided entirely, as will be seen, because there is no conceivable gain from them.

High-Risk Situations

A colleague recently told me about a case in his community. A man who had no family of his own and did not appear to date adults of either sex had become affiliated with a group that sponsored youth activities. He not only took kids on trips and activities but also welcomed them to his home at other times as well. He had several arcade machines that the kids could play for free. There were always teenage boys hanging around, and they were often invited to spend the night, even the weekend. But girls were never invited over.

This man was later indicted for child molestation—not surprisingly. But if this case seems obvious and extreme, it is well to remember that many parents dropped their kids off for the entire weekend who had never even met this man. I understand why men who have better cover than this one get away with it. They are hard to detect even with careful scrutiny. But I do not understand what these parents told themselves that would cause them to trust a man they'd never met who had an obvious proclivity toward spending time with children of a particular age and sex and who had no known adult relationships.

Simply put, be careful with men who involve themselves in youth activities and who do not have children of their own or children of that age. From church youth leaders to coaches to anyone who would befriend your child, notice if they have grown-up friends and partners. If they do not, be very cautious about leaving them alone with your child. In general, don't.

A friend called me recently. A young man has befriended the family of her son's best friend. The young man seems particularly taken with the children in the family. In fact, he seems to adore them, and he is over at the house, mostly playing with the children, almost daily. He does not appear to have any adult love interests, male or female. He has never been married, and he does not date. My friend has met him. He seems delightful, a bit immature perhaps, but really a nice guy. Did I think there was any problem with her leaving her own son alone with this man? Would I be concerned?

You bet I would. Would I be rude to him or refuse to go out to dinner with the family if he's along? Of course not. I have no proof at all that there is anything wrong with him. But would I quietly make sure my own children were never alone with him? Yes, because I know that he is in a high-risk category. I would do it for the same reason that I don't dive into pools that could hold hidden rocks. It only takes one.

I have since met this man. I like him. There is nothing about the way he talks or acts that suggests he is a child molester—which means nothing and changes nothing. I won't leave my children alone with him. "Liking" isn't enough for me to override what my head tells me. He is in a high-risk category, whether I like him or not.

Make no exceptions when considering a person's role. Priests, for example, have always qualified as a high-risk group. Professionals have seen them that way, most certainly since 1985 when the first of the major priest scandals broke in Louisiana. Looked at coldly, they have no known sexual relationships with adults, and they sometimes spend inordinate amounts of time with children. Of course, their celibacy is supposed to be because of a commitment to a higher calling, not a lack of interest in adult sex. And no doubt, it often is.

But turn the situation around and look at it from a pedophile's point of view. If he has no interest in adult sex, he is giving up nothing by "celibacy" and gaining a great deal: a socially acceptable excuse for having no adult love interests. In addition, the priesthood gives him an excuse for working with children as well as a position of great authority and guaranteed job security—traditionally that has been so regardless of whether he was caught molesting children.

For decades, the response of the church all over this country and abroad has been to move pedophilic priests from one parish to another and to continue to allow them access to children, a process that occurred as late as 1990.[2] This was a practice that absolutely did not escape the notice of pedophiles, even if it did the public. In addition, despite the fact that every single bishop had to know that the behavior was illegal, very few child molesting priests were ever turned over to authorities, another very strong perk from a pedophile's point of view.

As the press has amply reported, victims of abuse by clergy have traditionally been very effectively silenced. Historically, many have believed (or were convinced by others) that they could not attack the pedophile without attacking the church. Given all of these factors, the situation in the church for the past several decades has been the best of all possible worlds for pedophiles, and it was sure to draw them.

Pedophiles who seek such situations often focus much or all of their time or attention on children and have few or no adult social/sexual interests. In looking at such high-risk groups, note particularly anyone who focuses on a particular age and sex. Don't make exceptions because their role expects them to interact with children—remember they may have chosen the role for that reason. Nor should you make exceptions because many of the men in their group are not pedophiles and, in fact, may be unusually dedicated and responsible people. The concept of a "high-risk group" does not imply that everyone has the risk factor, only some.

Any situation that provides ideal conditions for pedophiles will draw them, and it will be very difficult to distinguish them from their nonpedophilic and entirely moral colleagues. Look at any arrangement in which pedophiles will thrive, and you will find pedophiles.

Although not as ideal as the priesthood, boarding schools, overnight camps, male choirs—any setting that puts groups of kids regularly together under the supervision and care of a "counselor" or other adult for overnight trips—will nonetheless draw pedophiles. Today I open the paper and learn that a nationally acclaimed children's choir, a choir that ran a residential program, was infiltrated by several pedophiles. A wealthy benefactor of the choir, who himself turned out to be a pedophile, recommended the others.

Recently I consulted on a legal case of a summer camp that inadvertently hired a pedophile as a camp counselor. The counselor was a man from another country, independently wealthy, who came over each summer to work in the camp. It was a clever move for a pedophile. No doubt he could have found camps in his own country, but molesting in a country where he did not live and where he was only present for a few months each year meant that if reported, he would have to be found in another country and extradited.

There are other signs to look for in addition to simply the presence of a setting that would draw pedophiles. If someone in a high-risk group seeks out your children, gives them small gifts, tries to see them outside the boundaries of the activity, then your suspicion should be doubled. Pedophiles rarely assault children violently. As we have seen, they more often worm their way into the child's affections and manipulate the child into having sex with them, using the child's naivety, loyalty, and trust. Giving gifts, showering attention and praise, taking kids for trips—all of these are part of the "worming in" or grooming process. The camp counselor mentioned above went so far as to visit the families of the children he was molesting when camp wasn't in session. He was so charming that he was even invited on vacation with some.

No one suspected him. The camp director even had her own son in his cabin. She thought his interest in the families and in spending time with the kids outside of camp was simply a reflection of what an ideal camp counselor he was. But it was also exactly the way a pedophile would act, and no one even considered that possibility.

Be especially careful if you are a single or divorced mom, and the child does not have a close relationship with his dad. Pedophiles will research children they are interested in to see who does or doesn't have a father in the home, who does or doesn't spend time with the father. Many of them believe kids without a father are more vulnerable. Of course, some such children are, and some aren't. Sometimes children without a father are more vulnerable only because the mother is so worried that the child doesn't have a male role model that she allows men out of the home to spend unusual amounts of time with her child. Most certainly, pedophiles will take advantage of that situation if they can find it.

With adult rape, as well, there are also high-risk and lower-risk circumstances. Someone you know well and have dated for a while is less likely to turn it out to be a rapist than a new acquaintance is, although it has certainly happened. The risk is higher with someone you are just beginning to date. This is so because many serial rapists use situations in which they can meet strangers to find victims. It is considerably easier to rape a woman they have lured to their apartment or another isolated setting than it is to take a chance on attacking someone on the street.

Also, it is much more difficult to prosecute date rape. Unless the violence produces overwhelming physical evidence, it comes down to "he said, she said." Even his DNA will not convict him. He will simply admit he had sex with his victim but insist it was consensual. After all, it was a "date," and she willingly went out with him. If he held a knife to her throat so that she could not fight without having her throat cut, there will not even be signs of a struggle. For these reasons date rape and certainly date rape drugs have become increasingly popular among serial rapists.

For such offenders, personal ads, dating services, fraternity parties, singles bars, and especially the Internet have become hunting grounds. The predators who use these situations will look and talk exactly like the men who are legitimately seeking a relationship. Many very violent men are gregarious, charming, and seemingly warm. Ted Bundy could have fit in well on any college campus.

If you decide to date a stranger, which frankly always involves some risk, at least take some basic safety precautions. First of all, if you've never met him before, then at least meet him with someone else present, if only for a moment. Have a friend with you at the restaurant or the bar when he arrives. Do not meet him at your home or apartment. If he is a rapist or potential stalker, you don't want him to know where you live. Tell someone where you're going and when you'll be back. Make sure someone else knows everything you know about him. And find a way to casually mention to him that someone else knows all about him. That will not necessarily protect you from being raped, but it will help insure you return afterward.

Remember that anyone is a stranger to you if you don't know his friends, the place he works, his life. If all you know about him comes from him—self-report through phone calls, emails, or dating service questionnaires—then all you know is what he claims. Find an excuse to call him at work. Look at a directory of his company. Make some attempt to verify at least that he has the identity he claims.

A colleague told me about a friend of his, a dentist who "fell in love" through the Internet. The picture he was sent was of a beautiful young woman who claimed to be the daughter of a Mafia don. The "relationship" progressed so far (without a single meeting) that a wedding was planned. Invitations went out, and his friends, including my colleague, were told the Mafia don would fly them all to Florida and back for the wedding. None of his friends felt easy about these developments—it all sounded too incredible—but the dentist was convinced and wouldn't listen to their concerns.

Finally, the day came when the dentist was to meet his bride, who was arriving in his town by bus. Friends noted it seemed an unusual way for a woman to travel who claimed to be able to charter private planes for her wedding, but the dentist didn't question it. She did arrive by bus. She was not the tall, thin, blond beauty in the photo but a very overweight, very short young woman with severe emotional problems. Needless to say, she was not the daughter of a Mafia don.

More than any other setting, the Internet permits deception. Correspondents can neither see nor hear each other and only "know" what the other person claims. Dating through the Internet is basically a variation on Russian roulette. It is the primary hunting ground for predators today. On it, anyone can pretend to be anything, a fact that has not escaped psychopathic attention. A rapist with three felony convictions can pretend to be a wealthy stock broker whose wife recently died. A forty-five-year-old man can successfully pretend to be a fourteen-year-old boy and draw in a fourteen-year-old girl who would not correspond knowingly with an adult male.

Research confirms the growing problem of predators approaching children on the Internet. A survey conducted by the Crimes Against Children Research Center at the University of New Hampshire found that one in five adolescents ages ten to seventeen who used the Internet had received a sexual solicitation in the preceding year, and one in thirty had received an aggressive solicitation.[3] An aggressive solicitation was defined as one in which the perpetrator made contact offline (through mail, phone, or in person) or attempted to persuade the child to engage in such offline contact.

Despite the fact that these numbers are alarming, it is highly likely that they are low, given the survey involved self-report. Knowing parents are extremely concerned about such approaches, it is likely many kids who were approached simply denied it for fear of losing access to the Internet.

What makes these figures particularly distressing, however, is that other research suggests children are not even in chat rooms all that much. A Kaiser Family Foundation survey of children ages eight to eighteen found that kids only averaged thirty-one minutes per day on the computer (although they spent 5.5 hours using some form of media). Eight- to thirteen-year-olds were the heaviest users, averaging more than an hour a day on the computer. Of that hour, however, only eleven minutes were spent in chat rooms. Yet the above data suggest that one in five was approached sexually.

Of particular concern is the fact that many of those who prey on kids are likely to be psychopaths. Psychopaths thrive on settings with conditions of anonymity, lawlessness, and lack of accountability. They do not do well in small towns because there is too much accountability: You cannot sell a car without a motor in a small town more than once. But psychopaths thrive in cities, the larger the better, and the Internet is now a very special kind of global city with all the conditions they require.

It is risky to let your children surf the Internet alone with no guidance and no software filters. Most certainly they should not be in chat rooms. And this includes teenagers. I doubt that there are very many children's chat rooms that do not have at least one sexual predator online at any given point. You can help your child find sites that are for children that do not permit interaction with strangers.

And there is an additional dark side to the Internet—aside from chat rooms and the predators who frequent them. It is incredibly easy to wander into a porn website, even a sadomasochistic one. Porn sites frequently take advantage of common misspellings or inaccurate web addresses to lure customers. For example, a website for teaching children about money was titled www.moneyopolis.com. A porn website was then set up as www.moneyopolis.org.[4] Children need supervision on the Internet. Software and/or parental guidance are necessary to find science and educational sites set up by reputable organizations that really are just for kids.

The issue with high-risk categories and high-risk situations isn't whether you know harm *will* occur in that setting but whether you know that there is a significant likelihood that harm *could* occur in such a setting. Look at any situation from the point of view of a rapist or child molester. If it looks ideal, count on them being there in numbers: Any setting in which they thrive will draw them. In dealing with such situations, remember that you don't have to be sure a man *is* a child molester to avoid leaving your child with him; you need to be pretty darn sure he isn't.

Low-Risk Situations

By definition, low-risk situations are where we want to be and where we want our kids to be. But there are some low-risk situations you can make even safer, and there are some you might want to avoid because—although they are low-risk—the gain from them is zero. For example, if you work with the public, you gain nothing from putting pictures of your children on your desk or in areas where the public will be, and it does involve some risk, however small. It only takes one person becoming sexually fixated on the smiling three-year-old for disaster to occur.

Some offenders have, indeed, become fixated on a particular child simply from seeing that child or a photo of him/her. An officer in a prison once told me the police came to his door in the middle of the night to tell him they had arrested a man outside his house. It was a neighbor who had been pacing back and forth outside his preschool daughter's window. The officer had been sleeping and had heard nothing, but another neighbor had gotten up to take the dog out, seen the intruder, and called the police. The police had come without lights or sirens and had watched quietly while the intruder paced back and forth, waiting to arrest him only when he opened the window to go in. If they had arrested him sooner, they would have only had him on a trespassing charge.

When they searched the offender's house, the police found approximately sixty pictures of the officer's little girl riding up and down the street on her bike. The offender had become obsessed with the child, had been watching her and taking photos of her for some time. He did not know this child or her father, and his obsession had developed just from seeing her. In this case, there was nothing the father could have done to prevent this fixation. But the same thing has happened with a picture on a desk at work. Keep your private life separate from dealing with casual coworkers and certainly from dealing with the public.

Carry a cell phone in a car. Being attacked in your car by a stranger is rare, but it does happen. I have treated women who have been run off the road by offenders and then raped, one in the middle of the day on a small town country road. I have talked to offenders who have deliberately caused minor wrecks in order to get their intended victim to stop and get out of the car. You are never alone with a cell phone. If there is trouble, you can always lock your doors, call the police, and wait for them to arrive. In my experience, some offenders see cell phones as a significant deterrent. I have known people to hold up a cell phone to prevent an attack and successfully back the offender off.

Likewise, it is not a bad idea to have a security system in your home, no matter where you live. Security systems screech and wail if someone tries to enter, then automatically dial the security service, which calls you back. If you don't answer with a password, they call the police. These systems are not that expensive. Admittedly, your home is a low-risk setting, at least for a stranger attack. But there is nothing wrong with making it lower still.

There is much talk of "panic rooms" right now, rooms that are built to be secure from intruders in which homeowners can hide until police come. However, the cost of such rooms makes them infeasible for most of us. In my opinion, they are excessive in any case, given the low probability of a home invasion and the fact that you have to get to them in a crisis, which isn't always possible. What is feasible, reasonable, and low-cost is to install deadbolts on several internal doors so that wherever you are in the house, you could lock yourself and your children inside. This would not necessarily stop an offender permanently: Doors can be shattered. But with a deadbolt, the offender would have to destroy the door to get inside, and that would take time—time you could use to escape through the window or use the phone, time for the police to arrive, even time just to yell.

Make a habit of keeping your cell phone in your room at night, not in your purse downstairs. I have known offenders, such as the one below, who cut the phone lines before coming in. The offender invaded a home looking for a fourteen-year-old boy he had planned to rape. He came in the house earlier in the day while someone was home and the door unlocked. He stole the keys from the woman's pocketbook while she was in another room. She heard a noise in the house and quickly realized her keys were gone. Nonetheless, she, her son, and her partner stayed there that night, an understandable decision—most of us are reluctant to leave our homes—but not a wise one.

The key thief came back that night, cut the phone lines, and calmly entered through the door. She and her partner heard him doing this and yelled at him to go away, but he continued. The two women and the son retreated to an upstairs bedroom with no deadbolt. The offender was so close behind them that part of his jacket got caught in the bedroom door when they slammed it. The offender couldn't get the cloth out and finally cut the piece of jacket off with the knife he was carrying for the assault.

The combined weight of the women was barely sufficient to stop the offender from breaking down the door. Desperate, the mother sent the teenage son out the second story window to climb down and get help. After he was gone, she yelled at the offender that her son had left and would be bringing the police. The offender broke off the attack suddenly and left. At the time, she assumed it was the knowledge that the police were coming that caused him to flee. More likely, it was the knowledge that his intended victim was gone.

When he was apprehended, it turned out all his known victims were young teenage boys, several of whom he had attacked after invading their homes. Had the mother not sent the son out, the intruder probably would have gotten through the door eventually. A deadbolt would have helped; a deadbolt and a cell phone would have stopped it.

If your keys are stolen, stay elsewhere until you can get the locks changed. Change your locks even if your keys are stolen in another city. A friend of mine and her husband drove to a city two hours from their home to spend the weekend, leaving their older teenage son at home. While in the city, her car keys were stolen. Before they returned home that weekend, their house was broken into (while their teenage son was home) by thieves using the keys. She still does not know how the thieves knew where she lived. Certainly, the address was not on the key ring.

A dog, if you can cope with one, is not a bad idea. I notice with interest that few homes in which abductions occur seem to have a dog. That is not an accident. Offenders who go in people's homes scout the terrain first. Even total strangers who have picked the child at random will drive by, back and forth, until they know who lives in the house with the child, what their hours are, and whether there is a dog.

I testified in a case in which the offender's most common modus operandus was to enter a house of a single mom early in the morning after she had left for work and before a thirteen-year-old boy left for school. In some, there was as little as a half an hour when the child was left alone. He did this several times, raping the child in the house each time. Obviously, it was not a coincidence that he was entering at exactly the point in time in which the age and sex child he preferred was home alone: Each house had been scouted carefully in advance. The offender's requirements were very particular: thirteen-year-old boy, single mom, child alone in the morning, and no dog.

Of course, an offender could kill a dog, but he would have to get to him first. Most dogs will bark at a stranger in the night long before the offender gets fully inside the house. While this won't help that much if the child is home alone and the phone lines are cut, it will certainly help in cases in which the child is abducted while the parents are sleeping.

You do not need an attack dog for this. Attack dogs are for professionals and pose too much risk to the children in the family, to their friends, and to the general public to be a good idea for amateur handlers. A poodle works just fine.

I learned the hard way the need for security against low-probability events—and about listening to a dog if you have one. You would think that professionals who work with and testify against criminals have the common sense to take precautions, but we are as prone to believing in positive illusions as anyone. Our own sense of personal invulnerability causes us to assume that attacks happen over there to someone else.

I was living in the country in New England while I worked at a nearby university. The road I lived on was a dead end and very isolated. Still, I had little fear of attack. At that time, the area had very little crime.

Because of my false sense of security (and my own positive illusions), I had taken no precautions. I had no security system and no deadbolts, and I often left the house unlocked. I had recently acquired a dog, but I couldn't let her outside much at night because she barked too much. I assumed the dog was simply a barker and tried to train her not to bark so much. Still, it should have told me something that she barked little in the day.

One evening in January I came home and found the woodstove burning wide open but still full of wood. There was no doubt an intruder had been in my home. Any wood I put in would have burned out in the ten hours I had been away, especially with the stove wide open. Besides the stove, he had also opened all the windows and left them open, not something I would have done in New England in January.

Suddenly, all the people I had testified against came back to me. There were some unsavory characters on that list, including sadists, and it would only take one with a taste for revenge. I had no thought at all that it could be connected to my personal life.

I called the local police, but they saw it as a petty case of vandalism at most. I was not so sure and asked a police chief from a neighboring town I knew to come and assess the situation. He was an experienced officer, someone who had worked organized crime in Boston before moving to the country. In addition, he had also grown up hunting and knew the woods.

The chief went all over my property, then told me someone had been watching the house. He showed me a path that had been made by walking back and forth between two viewing points, a path that was worn enough to suggest the visits had been going on for some time. One vantage point gave the intruder a view of the bathroom, another of the study where I worked. Unfortunately, I had made the viewing easy: I was out of sight of all neighbors and seldom closed the curtains.

When the dust settled, the overwhelmingly most likely candidate was not anyone I had dealt with professionally but rather someone from my personal life. I had a friend in graduate school who dated a cardiologist until he had a paranoid, psychotic break. When he became violent, she left him.

Later, police records showed, he had tried to kill several students in Madison, Wisconsin, by running his car off the road at them. He claimed he could "tell" they were gay and insisted they were making a pass at him (walking down the street while he was driving by). When the police searched his car, they found material in his car on serial killers, on how to kill people, and on which states had death penalties. Not the most reassuring reading material for a man who was floridly psychotic.

Through police files I learned he was a suspected serial killer of men. He kept turning up at the same time in the same areas where men disappeared and were later found murdered and mutilated. The autopsies suggested someone with medical experience, given the surgical precision with which various amputations were made on the victims.

I moved to town after the intruder got into my house, and shortly thereafter, this same man turned up at the home of a friend of mine in Boston, told her I had moved, and demanded to know where I had gone. She said (falsely) she had lost contact with me over the years. I had not seen this man for twenty years and had no idea he knew where I lived. For this and other reasons, I am relatively sure he is the man who got into my house.

The local police wrote up the incident, including the fact that he showed up at the house of a friend of mine asking where I had moved. I was standing in her home when the FBI called and asked about her contact with him. Apparently they were keeping tabs on him. She asked them if he was dangerous. There was a pause, and the agent suggested she never turn her back on him.

Truly, it was a one-in-a-million scenario. A man who could be a serial killer had found me, had stalked me silently, and had escalated to entering my house. It had nothing to do with all the trials or cases I had been in or the clients I had treated but instead was simply a random occurrence. Random and low probability maybe, but you can bet my security arrangements are a little better now.

Although the odds are very low that *you* will be attacked by a stranger in your home or that your child will be one of the very few abducted by nonfamily members each year, if you're that one, you really don't care what the odds were. Better to buy a few deadbolts. Better to add a security system. Better to keep your cell phone in your room at night. Better to get a dog. And better to pay attention if your dog starts barking in the night.

Choices

In protecting ourselves and our children, we should consider both detection and deflection. Detection, however, is very difficult, as discussed in Chapter 10. The things that will detect deception are subtle and not everyone can become proficient, no matter how hard he or she tries. It takes more than just knowledge: It takes spatial skills that allow someone to make minute distinctions in facial expressions and gesture. It takes the ability to pick up slight differences in rhythm and pitch and word usage. Some of us are naturally more attuned to words, others to visual clues, and some to neither. We have individual differences that make it possible or impossible to even use the information above.

Take my case, for example. I have barely enough spatial sense and visual memory to walk around safely. I cannot remember my friends' cars or recognize a face I have seen only a few times. The part of my brain that deals with space and shapes is likely a mass of shriveled neurons. For those of us with little spatial sense, detecting small differences in facial expression is pretty much impossible.

On the other hand, I'm not bad at statement analysis. The fact that

I study it is not the main thing—I study facial analysis too but still don't think I do it very well. But I can learn to analyze statements because most of my internal world is concerned with words. There are dialogues going on in my head all the time, sometimes between characters I've never met, embedded in stories I do not know. It is always the language I hear; I never see anybody. I even dream in dialogue, never pictures.

But even though I think I'm not bad at statement analysis, given what I know about deception and how hard it is to detect, I would not bet my children's safety on my or anyone's ability to detect it in any mode: words, face, body, or voice. It is deflection I am betting on.

And with deflection, there are choices to be made. The more we keep our children inside, the more we limit their contact with the outside world, the less likely it is that they will be molested. At the extreme, we could home school, keep our children away from all group sports and activities, and never let them go anywhere without escorting them. We might keep them safe from molestation, but few of us would think our children would benefit from such a cloistered childhood with so few opportunities for growth.

On the other hand, we could simply sign up for anything, assume anyone who has a ready smile is a good person, and send them off for overnights with any group that seems reputable. This is more the pattern in this country, but it too yields a fearful toll. As I've shown, even reputable groups are easily infiltrated by pedophiles, and the result, as we've seen earlier, is that a minimum of 20 percent of girls and 10 percent of boys in the United States are finding their way into the hands of child molesters.

It is a slider, this business of protecting our children. On the one extreme there would be few opportunities for our children but few opportunities for pedophiles as well. On the other extreme, there would be many opportunities for our children and many also for child molesters. Where you set the slider will determine how many opportunities your children have and how many molesters have.

Most of us want to be thoughtful about this, and we want to be somewhere in the middle. We do not want to deprive our children of everything in an effort to make them safe. But we also don't want to take risks with our children if we can accomplish the same thing with less risk. We don't want either extreme—no supervision or no opportunities.

Each parent's decision on these matters is a personal one. No book could or should try to make those choices for you. This book is simply a map of the terrain so that you can make those decisions knowing who the enemy is, how he thinks, and where he hides.

As for my decisions, look for me at basketball practice, on the soccer field, at Little League. I'm the woman sitting over there on the lawn chair with the baseball cap, the one at every practice, every game. I'm the one volunteering to help chaperone the overnights. I'm the parent whose children are in day camp, not overnight, the one who does not allow men without adult interests to shower favors on my children.

If I do my job right, my children's lives will be filled with so many opportunities and interests, they will not even notice what they're missing. The only one who will notice is that friendly, smiling, affable man with a secret life, the one at the sock hop, the one who's waiting for an opportunity that will never come.

NOTES

Introduction

1. Because the vast majority of offenders are male, male pronouns will be used more than female throughout this book when describing offenders in general.

2. The educational films include "Truth, Lies and Sex Offenders"; "Sadistic and Nonsadistic Sex Offenders: How They Think; What They Do"; and "Offenders Who Prey on Staff" (Newbury Park, Calif.: Sage Publications). The second and the third, however, are made primarily for professional audiences. Because of the content of the second film on sadists, particularly, I do not recommend it for the general public.

3. There are a few quotes that do not come from videotaped transcripts but rather come from interviews in which I took down the comments of the offenders and occasionally the victims verbatim on a computer. In any case, I did not rely on my memory for the exact quotes that are found throughout the book.

Chapter 1

1. Stevens, "Connoisseur of Chaos" (1982). Reprinted with permission.

2. All names are fictitious.

3. See, for example, Hamilton (1929); Kinsey et al. (1953); Landis (1940); Landis (1956); Terman (1951); Terman (1938).

4. See Hamilton (1929) and Landis (1956).

5. Abel et al. (1988); Abel et al. (1987); Abel et al. (1985); and Abel and Rouleau (1990).

6. Although more than twenty years old, this study is still the classic study on undetected offenses, largely because it had better guarantees on confidentiality than any study to date, and therefore it is likely that the offenders were less reluctant to reveal previously unknown offenses.

7. See, for example, Badgley (1984); Finkelhor et al. (1990); Russell (1984; 2000); Salter (1992); Stein et al. (1988); Wyatt and Powell (1988).

8. Badgley (1984); Salter (1992); Timnick (1985a; 1985b).

9. Russell (1984; 2000).

10. Koss (1993); and Koss and Harvey (1991).

11. Kilpatrick et al. (1992); Russell (2000).
12. Abma et al. (1997); Tjaden and Thoennes (1998).
13. Hindman and Peters (2001).

Chapter 2

1. See, for example, Ekman (1991; 1992).
2. See Gonzalez et al. (1993); Roesler and Wind (1994); Sauzier (1989); Smith et al. (2000); and Sorensen and Snow (1991) for studies on disclosure of child sexual abuse.

Chapter 3

1. Gratzer and Bradford (1995).
2. Warren et al. (1996).
3. De Becker (1997), p. 57.
4. See Ekman (1992) for a review.
5. Ibid.
6. Frank (1966).

Chapter 4

1. Knopp (1984), p. 9.
2. Herman (1981); Masson (1984); Rush (1980).
3. See, for example, Briere and Conte (1993); Brown et al. (1998); Elliot and Briere (1995); Feldman-Summers and Pope (1994); Pope and Tabachnick (1995); Saywitz et al. (1991); Scheflin and Brown (1996); Terr (1994); Van der Kolk et al. (1996); Williams (1992; 1994; 1995).
4. Abraham (1927), p. 50.
5. Ibid., p. 50.
6. Ibid., p. 51.
7. Ibid., pp. 52–53.
8. Ibid., p. 54.
9. Ibid., p. 57.
10. See, for example, Bender and Blau (1937); Bender and Grugett (1952); Henderson (1975; 1983); Lukianowicz (1972); Mohr et al. (1964); Revitch and Weiss (1962); Sloane and Karpinski (1942); Weiner (1962); Weiss et al. (1955).
11. Bender and Blau (1937, p. 514).
12. Ibid., p. 514.
13. Ibid., p. 514.
14. Gagnon (1965); Krieger et al. (1980); MacVicar (1979); Virkunnen (1975); Weiss et al. (1955).
15. Gagnon (1965).
16. Weiner (1962), p. 628.
17. Ibid., p. 614.

18. Yorukoglu and Kemph (1966).
19. Ibid., p. 123.
20. de Young (1982).
21. Rascovsky and Rascovsky (1950), p. 45.
22. DeMott (1980).
23. Virkunnen (1975), p. 179.
24. Ibid., p. 123.
25. Revitch and Weiss (1962), p. 78.
26. Ibid., p. 75.
27. Reported by the Associated Press (2002).
28. Carter (2002).
29. Rascovsky and Rascovsky (1950), p. 44.
30. Kaufman et al. (1954).
31. Gordan (1955).
32. Lustig et al. (1966), p. 34.
33. Ibid., p. 39.
34. Forward and Buck (1978).
35. Justice and Justice (1979).
36. Giarretto (1982), p. 19.
37. Tormes (1968).
38. Ibid., p. 27.
39. Trepper and Barrett (1989).
40. Ibid., p. 46.
41. Slovenko (1971), p. 158.
42. Ibid., p. 158.
43. Levine (2002a); Mirkin (1999); Rind et al. (1998).
44. Levine (2002a), p. 25.
45. American Psychiatric Association (2000).
46. Levine (2002a), p. 26.
47. See www.atsa.com/pubSoT.html for a description of the ATSA Standards and Guidelines.
48. Hanson et al. (2002).
49. See, for example, Furby et al. (1989) for an analysis of the impact of treatment that found older methods of treatment were not effective.
50. Levine (2002a), p. 26.
51. Hanson and Bussiere (1998). There was a second study that Levine cited: Alexander (1999). This study did not specify the follow-up time period used in the analysis. However, Dr. Alexander has stated that, "I don't question the findings from the Hanson meta-analysis that low reoffense rates are associated only with the first few years after release. Enough research has accumulated at this point to make it clear that long term reoffense rates are considerably higher than the 13% rate I found in my study, which I always saw as preliminary" (Alexander [2002]).
52. Doren (1998).
53. Prentky et al. (1997).

54. Hanson et al. (1993).
55. Levine (2002a), p. 86.
56. Phillips (1999).
57. National Campaign to Prevent Teen Pregnancy (2000).
58. Levine (2002a), p. 137.
59. Rind et al. (1998b).
60. Rind et al. (2001c).
61. Rind et al. (1998b), p. 34.
62. See, for example, Janoff-Bulman (1992); Janoff-Bulman and Timko (1987); and Taylor (1989).
63. Salter (1995).
64. Schlessinger (1999).
65. Both the North American Man Boy Love Association (NAMBLA) and the International Pedophile and Child Emancipation (IPCE) have praised the study. In fact, the IPCE has an entire section on their website devoted to research by Rind and colleagues.
66. Dallam (2002).
67. Dallam (2002); Dallam et al. (2001); Ondersma et al. (2001).
68. Rind et al. (2001a; 2001b); Rind et al. (1999; 2000; 2001c).
69. Rind et al. (1999).
70. Rind et al. (1999; 2000; 2001a).
71. "When Politics Clashes with Science" (2000).
72. *Paidika* (1987), pp. 2–3.
73. Underwager and Wakefield (1993).
74. Bauserman (1989); Rind (1995).
75. Rind et al. (1998a).
76. Bauserman (1990).
77. Finkelhor (1984); Mrazek (1985).
78. See, for example, Jumper (1995); Neuman et al. (1996); Oddone and Genuis (1996); Paolucci et al. (2001).
79. Boney-McCoy and Finkelhor (1995; 1996); Brown et al. (1999); Dinwiddie et al. (2000); Fergusson et al. (1996); Fleming et al. (1999); Johnson et al. (1999); Kendler et al. (2000); Mullen et al. (1993); Nelson et al. (2002); Stein et al. (1988).
80. Berliner and Conte (1990).
81. Ibid., p. 32.
82. Conte, Wolf, and Smith (1989).
83. Ibid., p. 296.
84. Ibid., p. 298.
85. Ibid., p. 298.
86. Ibid., p. 298.
87. Elliott et al. (1995), p. 584.
88. Mirkin (1999).
89. Levine (2002a), p. 23.
90. Levine (2002b).

91. Levine (2002a), p. 23.
92. Lustig et al. (1966), p. 34.
93. Rascovsky and Rascovsky (1950), p. 44.
94. Gebhard (1965).
95. Swanson (1968), p. 681.
96. Freund et al. (1972).
97. Groth (1982).
98. Lanyon (1986).
99. Eldridge (1995).
100. See, for example, Garlick et al. (1996); Nichols and Molinder (1996).
101. Knopp (1984).
102. Hindman and Peters (2001).
103. The immunity was conditional and dependent on the offender success-fully completing five years of treatment and not reoffending.
104. See, for example, Ansley (1997).
105. Hislop (2001).
106. Motiuk and Belcourt (1996).
107. Davin, Hislop, and Dunbar (1999); Matthews et al. (1989); Rosencrans (1997); Saradjian (1996).
108. Rosencrans (1997), p. 29.
109. Ibid., p. 111.
110. Saradjian (1996), p. 36.
111. Ibid.
112. Ibid.
113. Rosencrans (1997).

Chapter 5

1. Kilpatrick et al. (1992); Russell (2000).
2. Bureau of Justice Statistics (2000).
3. Ibid.
4. Saunders (2001).
5. Epperson (2000).
6. The basis for this typology comes from the work of Knight (1999).
7. Ibid.

Chapter 6

1. Abel et al. (1981), p. 133.
2. Ibid.
3. Groth (1979).
4. Fine (1990), p. 168.
5. Gelinas (1992).
6. Langevin (1990).
7. Abel et al. (1977). Sexual arousal was measured by the plethysmograph,

which consists of a small, lightweight aluminum gauge that the offender places on his penis while in a room alone. Wires are attached to the gauge and go out of the room to a computer in another room. The computer measures the amount of erection the offender has in response to stories of sexual interactions with different age partners and with different degrees of violence.

8. American Psychiatric Association (2000).

9. Groth (1979), p. 56.

10. Warren et al. (1996).

11. Heilbroner (1993), p. 147.

12. De Young (1982), p. 125.

13. Michaud and Aynesworth (1989).

14. Ibid., p. 188.

15. Ibid., p. 135.

16. Heilbroner (1993), p. 148.

17. Warren et al. (1996).

18. Gratzer and Bradford (1995).

19. Warren et al. (1996).

20. Hazelwood et al. (1993).

21. Michaud (1994), p. 176.

Chapter 7

1. Hare (1996).

2. Babiak (2000).

3. Forth and Burke (1998).

4. Hemphill et al. (1998); Serin (1996).

5. Hare et al. (1988); Harris et al. (1991).

6. Hemphill (1998).

7. Babiak (2000).

8. Lykken (1995), p. 120.

9. Cleckley (1976); Plutarch (1992).

10. Plutarch (1992), p. 259.

11. Plutarch (1992), p. 261.

12. Durant (1939), p. 445.

13. Plutarch (1992), p. 261.

14. Ibid., p. 260.

15. Ibid., p. 264.

16. Ibid., p. 277.

17. Ibid., p. 270.

18. Ibid., p. 275.

19. Ibid., p. 275.

20. Buchanan (1948), p. 184.

21. Ibid., p. 180.

22. Ibid., p. 181.

Chapter 8

1. Allen and Bosta (1981).
2. Cialdini (1993).
3. Ibid.
4. Regan (1971).

Chapter 9

1. Stevens, "The Man with the Blue Guitar" (1982). Reprinted with permission.
2. See, for example, Matlin and Stang (1978); Taylor (1989; 1998); Taylor and Brown (1988); Tiger (1979).
3. Taylor (1989).
4. Taylor et al. (submitted for publication).
5. Johnson (1937). The fact that research on this issue stretches from 1937 to the present day only underscores the robustness of this phenomenon. Much has changed in the world in the past sixty-five years, but not, apparently, our collective illusions about ourselves and the world.
6. Alicke (1985); Brown (1986).
7. Campbell (1986); Lewicki (1984).
8. Campbell (1986); Marks (1984).
9. See, for example, DePaulo et al. (1985); Ekman (1991; 1992); Kraut (1980); Zuckerman et al. (1981).
10. For example, DePaulo and Pfeifer (1986); Ekman (1991); Kohnken (1987); Kraut and Poe (1980).
11. Kraut and Poe (1980).
12. DePaulo and Pfeifer (1986).
13. Kohnken (1987).
14. Ekman (1991).
15. Ekman claims that 53 percent scored from 70 to 100 percent, which he defines as above-chance levels. However, a subsequent analysis by Nickerson and Hammond (1993) suggested that Ekman made a statistical error and was incorrect in considering 7 out of 10 significantly higher than chance. Statistically, in this instance only 8 out of 10 or above would actually be higher than chance. Only 29 percent of the Secret Service performed at this level.
16. DePaulo and Pfeifer (1986).
17. Kohnken (1987).
18. Ekman (1991).
19. Gilbert (1991); Gilbert et al. (1990; 1993).
20. Arkes et al. (1989; 1991); Begg et al. (1985); Hasher et al. (1977).
21. Gerrig and Prentice (1991); Gilbert et al. (1990); Wegner et al. (1994).
22. Gilbert et al. (1990; 1993).
23. De Becker (1997).
24. Ibid., p. 5.

25. DePaulo (1981); DePaulo et al. (1980); Goleman (1985); Rosenthal and DePaulo (1979); Zuckerman et al. (1981).
26. Goleman (1985).
27. Ibid., p. 221.
28. Henslin (1967).
29. Langer (1975).
30. Brison (2001).
31. Having worked with rapists for many years, I do not subscribe to the notion that what victims wear influences whether they are attacked. I mention her clothing only because I am aware that those who blame victims for assaults often believe this.
32. Scheppele and Bart (1983).
33. Dyer (2001).
34. Dyer (2001), p. 17.
35. Lamott (1994).
36. Norris (1992).
37. Norris (1992).
38. Dillard (1974), pp. 6–7.
39. Matlin and Stang (1978).
40. Lerner (1980).
41. Lerner (1980), p. 4.
42. Miller and Tompkins (1977), p. 86.
43. Lerner (1980), p. 120.
44. Reed et al. (1994; 1999); Taylor et al. (2000).
45. Taylor et al. (submitted for publication).
46. Colvin and Block (1994); Colvin et al. (1995); John and Robbins (1994); Paulhus (1998); Shedler et al. (1993).
47. John and Robbins (1994).
48. Colvin et al. (1995).
49. Colvin et al. (1995); Shedler et al. (1993).
50. Tiger (1979), p. 283.
51. Janoff-Bulman (1992).
52. Miller and Tompkins (1977); Terr (1990).
53. Terr (1990).
54. Terr (1985a; 1985b; 1990).
55. Terr (1990).
56. Terr (1985b), p. 820.
57. Terr (1990) p. 31.
58. Famularo et al. (1990).
59. Janoff-Bulman (1992).
60. Tiger (1979), p. 69.
61. Spiegel (1990), p. 251.
62. Didion (1979), pp. 11–13.
63. Dillard (1974), p. 177.
64. Salter (1995).

Chapter 10

1. Stevens, "The Snow Man" (1982). Reprinted with permission.
2. Janoff-Bulman (1992), p. 24.
3. Gollwizer and Kinney (1989); Taylor and Gollwizer (1995).
4. Warren et al. (1996).
5. Eldridge (1995), pp. 138–139.
6. Ekman (1992).
7. Ekman (1992), p. 141.
8. Abel et al. (1985; 1987); Groth et al. (1982); Russell (1984); Weinrott and Saylor (1991).
9. Ekman (1992).
10. See Ansley (1997) for a review of polygraph studies.
11. Ekman (1989).
12. Forte (1986).
13. Ekman (1989).
14. Ekman (1992).
15. Ibid.
16. Ibid.
17. Ekman (1992); Ekman and Rosenberg (1997).
18. Ekman (1992).
19. Ibid.
20. Ekman (1982).
21. Computerized versions of FACS are being developed and normed but are not yet available for clinical use. See Cohn et al. (1999; 2001); Tian et al. (2000; 2001).
22. Rudacille (1992; 1994) looked at one hundred people accused of a crime, of whom fifty-two failed a polygraph and forty-eight passed it. As added insurance that his groups were truly genuine groups of people lying and people truth-telling, he looked for outside collaboration. Of the people who failed the polygraph, 94 percent of the time outside collaboration indicated they were, indeed, lying: For example, either they eventually confessed or were convicted. Of the people who passed the polygraph, 73 percent of the time there was eventually evidence that they were telling the truth: For example, someone else was convicted or confessed.The differences in speech were striking, particularly in regard to evasive answers. In the interviews with the forty-eight people telling the truth, evasive answers were given at an average rate of one per interview, for a total of forty-eight evasions. By contrast, the fifty-two interviews with the liars produced three hundred twenty-two evasive answers, or more than six times as many. The detail made the differences even more striking. In the case of the liars, 95 percent of the time, the question they evaded was about the crime. In the case of the truth-tellers, 80 percent of the time the evasion was *not* about the crime but about some other issue that came up in the interview.
23. Rudacille (1994).
24. Information on Sapir's work is available from www.lsiscan.com. It is not clear that Rudacille's work and Sapir's work are actually separate systems. Sapir

points out that Rudacille took his course on statement analysis in 1990 and feels Rudacille's work is simply an extension of principles he developed (Sapir, personal communication, September 8, 2001).

25. The single study was by Driscoll (1994) and had a sample size of thirty subjects (twenty-five male and five female), all of whom were accused of a crime. Based on evidence, convictions, confessions, polygraph, and other evidence, eleven people were considered likely innocent and nineteen likely guilty. Sapir's techniques were then used to analyze the statements of the thirty suspects. Of the eleven ultimately thought innocent, eight tested truthful on Sapir's system whereas three showed indications of deception. In one of those, however, the evidence of deception was not around the crime but around a second issue about which he was interviewed. In the case of those ultimately thought guilty, all but one tested deceptive on Sapir's system. The one who did not test deceptive only wrote three lines and refused to write more. It is not likely or even to be expected that statement analysis would work on such a small sample of speech. Thus, although the system is certainly not perfect, it did reliably detect deception and truthfulness in most subjects. Of the different indicators of deception, the one that was most accurate was outright denial (or failure to deny), which distinguished between the two groups two-thirds of the time.

26. Some readers may be familiar with a methodology called Statement Validity Assessment. Statement Validity Assessment was originally developed in Germany for use in the court system (Undeutsch [1989]). A modification of it, Criterion Based Content Analysis, has been used in this country primarily with child victims of sexual abuse (Steller and Koehnken [1990]). Sapir and Rudacille's systems were not based on and use different principles than either Statement Validity Analysis or Criterion Based Content Analysis.

27. Sapir has a series of workshop manuals that give more information. Of particular interest is a compilation of Sapir's newsletters, which can be ordered from him directly. In them he has analyses of, for example, interviews with Jeffrey McDonald (the Green Beret killer), testimony in the William Kennedy Smith rape trial, statements of Clarence Thomas and Anita Hill, and many other public cases.

28. Henderson (1994).

29. A complete retelling of the Susan Smith case, including this and other quotations, is available from www.crimelibrary.com/fillicide/smith.

30. Ibid.

Chapter 11

1. Nack and Yaeger (1999).
2. Rezendes and Carroll (2002).
3. Finkelhor et al. (2001).
4. Thornburg and Lin (in press).

BIBLIOGRAPHY

Abel, G. G., and J. L. Rouleau (1990). "The nature and extent of sexual assault." In W. L. Marshall, D. R. Laws, and H. E. Barbaree, *Handbook of Sexual Assault: Issues, Theories and Treatment of the Offender.* New York: Plenum Press. 9–21.

Abel, G. G., et al. (1977). "The components of rapists' sexual arousal." *Archives of General Psychiatry* 34(8): 895–903.

_____ (1981). "Identifying dangerous child molesters." In R. Stuart, *Violent Behavior: Social Learning Approaches to Prediction, Management, and Treatment.* New York: Brunner/Mazel. 117–131.

_____ (1985). "Sexual offenders: Results of assessment and recommendations for treatment." In M. H. Ben-Aron, S. J. Huckle, and C. D. Webster, *Clinical Criminology: The Assessment and Treatment of Criminal Behavior.* Toronto: M & M Graphic Ltd. 191–205.

_____ (1987). "Self-reported sex crimes of nonincarcerated paraphiliacs." *Journal of Interpersonal Violence* 2(1): 3–25.

_____ (1988). "Multiple paraphilic diagnoses among sex offenders." *Bulletin of the American Academy of Psychiatry and the Law* 16(2): 153–168.

Abma, J., et al. (1997). "Fertility, family planning, and women's health: New data from the 1995 National Survey of Family Growth, National Center for Health Statistics." *Vital and Health Statistics* 23(19).

Abraham, K. (1927). "The experiencing of sexual traumas as a form of sexual activity." *Selected Papers.* London: Hogarth. 47–62.

Alexander, M. (1999). "Sexual offender treatment efficacy revisited." *Sexual Abuse: A Journal of Research and Treatment* 11(2): 101–116.

_____ (2002, June 27). Personal communication. Madison, Wisc.

Alicke, M. D. (1985). "Global self-evaluation as determined by the desirability and controllability of trait adjectives." *Journal of Personality and Social Psychology* 49: 1621–1630.

Allen, B., and D. Bosta (1981). *Games Criminals Play.* Sacramento, Calif.: Rae John Publishers.

American Psychiatric Association (2000). *Diagnostic and Statistical Manual of Mental Disorders.* Washington, D.C.: American Psychiatric Association.

Ansley, N. (1997). "The validity and reliability of polygraph testing." *Polygraph* 26(4): 215–239.

Arkes, H. R., et al. (1989). "The generality of the relation between familiarity and judged validity." *Journal of Behavioral Decision Making* 2: 81–94.

_____ (1991). "Determinants of judged validity." *Journal of Experimental Social Psychology* 27: 576–605.

Associated Press (2002, April 29). "Court documents filed by Cardinal Law say negligence by boy, parents contributed to alleged sexual abuse."

Babiak, P. (2000). "Psychopathic manipulation at work." In C. B. Gacono, *The Clinical and Forensic Assessment of Psychopathy.* Mahwah, NJ: Lawrence Erlbaum. 287–311.

Badgley, R. F. (1984). *Sexual Offenses Against Children: Report of the Committee on Sexual Offenses Against Children and Youths.* Ottawa: Canadian Government Publishing Centre.

Bauserman, R. (1989). "Man-boy sexual relationships in a cross-cultural perspective." *Paidika: The Journal of Paedophilia* 2(5): 28–40.

_____ (1990). "Objectivity and ideology: Criticism of Theo Sandfort's research on man-boy relations." *Journal of Homosexuality* 20: 297–312.

Begg, L., et al. (1985). "On believing what we remember." *Canadian Journal of Behavioral Science* 17: 199–214.

Bender, L., and A. Blau (1937). "The reaction of children to sexual relations with adults." *American Journal of Orthopsychiatry* 7: 500–518.

Bender, L., and A. E. Grugett (1952). "A follow-up report on children who had atypical sexual experience." *American Journal of Orthopsychiatry* 22: 825–837.

Berliner, L., and J. R. Conte (1990). "The process of victimization: The victims' perspective." *Child Abuse and Neglect: The International Journal* 14(1): 29–40.

Boney-McCoy, S., and D. Finkelhor (1995). "Psychosocial sequelae of violent victimization in a national youth sample." *Journal of Consulting and Clinical Psychology* 63: 726–736.

_____ (1996). "Is youth victimization related to trauma symptoms and depression after controlling for prior symptoms and family relationships? A longitudinal, prospective study." *Journal of Consulting and Clinical Psychology* 64: 1406–1416.

Briere, J. N., and J. R. Conte (1993). "Self-reported amnesia for abuse in adults molested as children." *Journal of Traumatic Stress* 6(1): 21–31.

Brison, S. J. (2001). *Aftermath: Violence and the Remaking of a Self.* Princeton: Princeton University Press.

Brown, D., et al. (1998). *Memory, Trauma, Treatment, and the Law.* New York: W. W. Norton.

Brown, J. D. (1986). "Evaluations of self and others: Self-enhancement biases in social judgment." *Social Cognition* 4: 353–376.

Brown, J. D., et al. (1999). "Childhood abuse and neglect. Specificity of effects on adolescent and young adult depression and suicidality." *Journal of the American Academy of Child and Adolescent Psychiatry* 38(12): 1490–1496.

Buchanan, S., ed. (1948). *The Portable Plato.* New York: Viking Press.

Bureau of Justice Statistics, U.S. Department of Justice (2000). "National Crime Victimization Survey 2000."

Campbell, J. D. (1986). "Similarity and uniqueness: The effects of attribute type, relevance, and individual differences in self-esteem and depression." *Journal of Personality and Social Psychology* 50: 181–294.

Carter, C. J. (2002, June 10). "Little ado over teacher-pupil sex cases." *Boston Globe.*

Cialdini, R. B. (1993). *Influence.* New York: HarperCollins.

Cleckley, H. (1976). *The Mask of Sanity.* St. Louis, Mo.: C. V. Mosby.

Cohn, J., et al. (2001). "A comparative study of alternative FACS coding algorithms." Robotics Institute, Carnegie Mellon University.

Cohn, J. F., et al. (1999). "Automated face analysis by feature point tracking has high concurrent validity with manual FACS coding." *Psychophysiology* 36: 35–43.

Colvin, C. R., and J. Block (1994). "Do positive illusions foster mental health? An examination of the Taylor and Brown formulation." *Psychological Bulletin* 116(1): 3–20.

Colvin, C. R., et al. (1995). "Overly positive self-evaluations and personality: Negative implications for mental health." *Journal of Personality and Social Psychology* 68: 1152–1162.

Conte, J. R., et al. (1989). "What sexual offenders tell us about prevention strategies." *Child Abuse and Neglect: The International Journal* 13(2): 293–301.

Dallam, S. J. (2002). "Science or propaganda? An examination of Rind, Tromovitch and Bauserman (1998)." *Journal of Child Sexual Abuse* 9(3/4): 109–134.

Dallam, S. J., et al. (2001). "The effects of child sexual abuse: Comment on Rind, Tromovitch, and Bauserman (1998)." *Psychological Bulletin* 127(6): 715–733.

Davin, P. A., et al. (1999). *Female Sexual Abusers.* Brandon, Vt.: Safer Society Press.

De Becker, G. (1997). *The Gift of Fear.* Boston: Little, Brown.

DeMott, B. (1980). "The pro-incest lobby." *Psychology Today* 13(10): 11–12, 15–16.

DePaulo, B. (1981). "Success at detecting deception: Liability or skill." *Annals of the New York Academy of Science* 364: 245–255.

DePaulo, B. M., and R. L. Pfeifer (1986). "On-the-job experience and skill at detecting deception." *Journal of Applied Social Psychology* 16: 249–267.

DePaulo, B. M., et al. (1980). "Humans as lie detectors." *Journal of Communications* 30: 129–139.

————— (1985). *Deceiving and Detecting Deceit. The Self and Social Life.* New York: McGraw-Hill. 323–370.

de Young, M. (1982). *The Sexual Victimization of Children.* Jefferson, N.C.: McFarland.

Didion, J. (1979). *The White Album.* New York: Simon & Schuster.

Dillard, A. (1974). *Pilgrim at Tinker Creek.* New York: Bantam Books.

Dinwiddie, S., et al. (2000). "Early sexual abuse and lifetime psychopathology: A co-twin-control study." *Psychological Medicine* 30: 41–52.

Doren, D. M. (1998). "Recidivism base rates, predictions of sex offender recidivism and the 'sexual predator' commitment laws." *Behavioral Sciences and the Law* 16: 97–114.

Driscoll, L. N. (1994). "A validity assessment of written statements from suspects in criminal investigations using the SCAN technique." Paper presented at the meeting of the Academy of Criminal Justice Sciences, Chicago, Ill.

Durant, W. (1939). *The Life of Greece: The Story of Civilization.* New York: MJF Books.

Dyer, W. W. (2001). *There's a Spiritual Solution to Every Problem.* New York: HarperCollins.

Ekman, P. (1982). "Methods for measuring facial action." In K. R. Scherer and P. Ekman, *Handbook of Methods in Nonverbal Behavioral Research.* Cambridge: Cambridge University Press. 45–90.

_____ (1989). "Why lies fail and what behaviors betray a lie." In J. C. Yuille, *Credibility Assessment.* Boston: Kluwer Academic.

_____ (1991). "Who can catch a liar?" *American Psychologist* 46: 913–920.

_____ (1992). *Telling Lies.* New York: W. W. Norton.

Ekman, P., and E. Rosenberg (1997). *What the Face Reveals.* New York: Oxford University Press.

Eldridge, H. (1995). "Apology and forgiveness." In A. C. Salter, *Transforming Trauma: A Guide to Understanding and Treating Adult Survivors of Child Sexual Abuse.* Newbury Park, Calif.: Sage.

Elliot, D. M., and J. Briere (1995). "Posttraumatic stress associated with delayed recall of sexual abuse: A general population study." *Journal of Traumatic Stress* 8: 629–647.

Elliott, M., et al. (1995). "Child sexual abuse prevention: What offenders tell us." *Child Abuse and Neglect: The International Journal* 19: 579–594.

Epperson, D. (2000). "Minnesota Sex Offense Screening Tool—Revised." Presented at Sinclair Seminars Sex Offender Re-Offense Risk Prediction, Madison, Wisc.

Famularo, R., et al. (1990). "Symptom differences in acute and chronic presentation of childhood post-traumatic stress disorder." *Child Abuse and Neglect: The International Journal* 14(3): 439–444.

Feldman-Summers, S., and K. S. Pope (1994). "The experience of 'forgetting' childhood abuse: A national survey of psychologists." *Journal of Consulting and Clinical Psychology* 62(3): 636–639.

Fergusson, D. M., et al. (1996). "Childhood sexual abuse and psychiatric disorder in young adulthood: II. Psychiatric outcomes of childhood sexual abuse." *Journal of the American Academy of Child and Adolescent Psychiatry* 34: 1365–1374.

Fine, C. G. (1990). "The cognitive sequelae of incest." In R. P. Kluft, *Incest Related Syndromes of Adult Psychopathology.* Washington, D.C.: American Psychiatric Press. 161–182.

Finkelhor, D. (1984). "Youths not always victims in man-boy sex, survey reveals." *Forum* 14(1): 8–9.

Finkelhor, D., et al. (1990). "Sexual abuse in a national survey of adult men and women: Prevalence, characteristics, and risk factors." *Child Abuse and Neglect: The International Journal* 14(1): 19–28.

_____ (2001). Youth Internet Safety Survey. University of New Hampshire, Crimes Against Children Research Center.

Fleming, J., et al. (1999). "The long-term impact of childhood sexual abuse in Australian women." *Child Abuse and Neglect: The International Journal* 23: 145–159.

Forte, S. (1986). *Read the Dealer.* Berkeley, Calif.: RGA.

Forth, A. E., and H. C. Burke (1998). "Psychopathy in adolescence: Assessment, violence, and developmental precursors." In D. J. Cooke, A. E. Forth, and R. D. Hare, *Psychopathy: Theory, Research and Implications for Society.* Dordrecht, The Netherlands: Kluwer Academic. 205–229.

Forward, S., and C. Buck (1978). *Betrayal of Innocence: Incest and Its Devastation.* New York: J. P. Tarcher.

Frank, G. (1966). *The Boston Strangler.* New York: New American Library.

Freund, K., et al. (1972). "The female child as a surrogate object." *Archives of Sexual Behavior* 2(2): 119–133.

Furby, L., et al. (1989). "Sex offender recidivism: A review." *Psychological Bulletin* 105(1): 3–30.

Gagnon, J. H. (1965). "Female child victims of sex offense." *Social Problems* 13(2): 176–192.

Garlick, I., et al. (1996). "Intimacy deficits and attribution of blame among sex offenders." *Legal and Criminological Psychology* 1: 251–258.

Gebhard, P. H., et al. (1965). *Sex Offenders: An Analysis of Types.* New York: Harper and Row.

Gelinas, D. (1992). "On being the chosen one in a malevolent family environment" Paper presented at the conference Psychological Trauma: Maturational Processes and Therapeutic Interventions, Boston, Mass.

Gerrig, R. J., and D. A. Prentice (1991). "The representation of fictional information." *Psychological Science* 2: 336–340.

Giarretto, H. (1982). *Integrated Treatment of Child Sexual Abuse.* Palo Alto, Calif.: Science and Behavior Books.

Gilbert, D. T. (1991). "How mental systems believe." *American Psychologist* 46: 107–119.

Gilbert, D. T., et al. (1990). "Believing the unbelievable: Some problem in the rejection of false information." *Journal of Personality and Social Psychology* 59(4): 601–613.

Gilbert, D. T., et al. (1993). "You can't not believe everything you read." *Journal of Personality and Social Psychology* 65(2): 221–233.

Goleman, D. (1985). *Vital Lies, Simple Truths: The Psychology of Self-Deception.* New York: Simon & Schuster.

Gollwizer, P. M., and R. F. Kinney (1989). "Effects of deliberative and implemental mind-sets on illusion of control." *Journal of Personality and Social Psychology* 56: 531–542.

Gonzalez, L. S., et al. (1993). "Children's patterns of disclosures and recantations of sexual and ritualistic abuse allegations in psychotherapy." *Child Abuse and Neglect* 17(2): 281–289.

Gordan, L. (1955). "Incest as revenge against the pre-Oedipal mother." *Psychoanalytic Review* 42: 284–292.

Gratzer, T., and J. M. W. Bradford (1995). "Offender and offense characteristics of sexual sadists: A comparative study." *Journal of Forensic Sciences* 40(3): 450–455.

Groth, A. N. (1979). *Men Who Rape: The Psychology of the Offender.* New York: Plenum Press.

Groth, A. N., et al. (1982). "Undetected recidivism among rapists and child molesters." *Crime and Delinquency* 28(3): 450–458.

Groth, N. (1982). "The incest offender." In S. Sgroi, *Handbook of Clinical Intervention in Child Sexual Abuse.* Lexington, Mass.: Lexington Books. 215–239.

Hamilton, G. V. (1929). *A Research in Marriage.* New York: Albert & Charles Boni.

Hanson, R. K., et al. (1993). "Long-term recidivism of child molesters." *Journal of Consulting and Clinical Psychology* 61(4): 646–652.

Hanson, R. K., and M. T. Bussiere (1998). "Predicting relapse: A meta-analysis of sexual offender recidivism studies." *Journal of Consulting and Clinical Psychology* 66(2): 348–362.

Hanson, R. K., et al. (2002). "First report of the Collaborative Outcome Data Project on the Effectiveness of Psychological Treatment for Sex Offenders." *Sexual Abuse: A Journal of Research and Treatment* 14(2): 169–194.

Hare, R. D. (1996). "Psychopathy: A clinical construct whose time has come." *Criminal Justice and Behavior* 23(1): 25–54.

Hare, R. D., et al. (1988). "Male psychopaths and their criminal careers." *Journal of Consulting and Clinical Psychology* 56: 710–714.

Harris, G. T., et al. (1991). "Psychopathy and violent recidivism." *Law & Human Behavior* 15(6): 625–637.

Hasher, L., et al. (1977). "Frequency and the conference of referential validity." *Journal of Verbal Learning and Verbal Behavior* 16: 107–112.

Hazelwood, R., et al. (1993). "Compliant victims of the sexual sadist." *Australian Family Physician* 22(4): 474–479.

Heilbroner, D. (1993). "Serial murder and sexual repression." *Playboy* 78: 147–150.

Hemphill, J. F., et al. (1998). "Psychopathy and recidivism: A review." *Legal and Criminological Psychology* 3: 139–170.

Henderson, D. J. (1975). "Incest." In A. M. Freedman, H. I. Kaplan, and B. J. Sadock, *Comprehensive Textbook of Psychiatry.* Baltimore: Williams and Wilkins. 1530–1539.

Henderson, G. (1994, October 27). "Children's kidnapper still eludes authorities." *Spartanburg, South Carolina, Herald-Journal.*

Henderson, J. (1983). "Is incest harmful?" *Canadian Journal of Psychiatry* 28(1): 34–40.

Henslin, J. M. (1967). "Craps and magic." *American Journal of Sociology* 73: 316–330.

Herman, J. L. (1981). *Father-Daughter Incest.* Cambridge, Mass.: Harvard University Press.

Hindman, J., and J. Peters (2001). "Polygraph testing leads to better understanding adult and juvenile sex offenders." *Federal Probation* 65(3): 8–15.

Hislop, J. (2001). *Female Sex Offenders.* Ravendale, Wash.: Issues Press.

Janoff-Bulman, R. (1992). *Shattered Assumptions: Towards a New Psychology of Trauma.* New York: Free Press.

Janoff-Bulman, R., and C. Timko (1987). "Coping with traumatic life events: The role of denial in light of people's assumptive worlds." In C. R. Snyder and C. Ford, *Coping with Negative Life Events: Clinical and Social Psychological Perspectives.* New York: Plenum Press.

John, O. P., and R. W. Robbins (1994). "Accuracy and bias in self-perception: Individual differences in self-enhancement and the role of narcissism." *Journal of Personality and Social Psychology* 66: 206–219.

Johnson, J. G., et al. (1999). "Childhood maltreatment increases risk for personality disorders during early adulthood." *Archives of General Psychiatry* 56: 600–606.

Johnson, W. B. (1937). "Euphoric and depressed mood in normal subjects." *Character and Personality* 6: 79–98.

Jumper, S. A. (1995). "A meta-analysis of the relationship of child sexual abuse to adult psychological adjustment." *Child Abuse and Neglect: The International Journal* 19: 715–728.

Justice, B., and R. Justice (1979). *The Broken Taboo.* New York: Human Services.

Kanade, T., et al. (2000). Comprehensive database for facial expression analysis. *Proceedings of the 4th IEEE International Conference on Automatic Face and Gesture Recognition,* Grenoble, France.

Kaufman, I., et al. (1954). "The family constellation and overt incestuous relations between father and daughter." *American Journal of Orthopsychiatry* 24: 266–279.

Kendler, K. S., et al. (2000). "Childhood sexual abuse and adult psychiatric and substance use disorders in women: An epidemiological and cotwin control analysis." *Archives of General Psychiatry* 57: 953–959.

Kilpatrick, D. G., et al. (1992). *Rape in America: A Report to the Nation.* Arlington, Va.: National Victim's Center.

Kinsey, A. C., et al. (1953). *Sexual Behavior in the Human Female.* Philadelphia: Saunders.

Knight, R. A. (1999). "Validation of a typology for rapists." *Journal of Interpersonal Violence* 14(3): 330.

Knopp, F. H. (1984). *Retraining Adult Sex Offenders: Methods and Models.* Orwell, Vt.: Safer Society Press.

Kohnken, G. (1987). "Training police officers to detect deceptive eyewitness statements: Does it work." *Social Behaviour* 2: 1–17.

Koss, M. P. (1993). "Detecting the scope of rape: A review of prevalence research methods." *Journal of Interpersonal Violence* 8(2): 198–222.

Koss, M. P., and M. R. Harvey (1991). *The Rape Victim*. Newbury Park, Calif.: Sage.

Kraut, R. E. (1980). "Humans as lie detectors: Some second thoughts." *Journal of Communication* 30: 209–216.

Kraut, R. E., and D. Poe (1980). "On the line: The deception judgments of customs inspectors and laymen." *Journal of Personality and Social Psychology* 39: 784–798.

Krieger, M. J., et al. (1980). "Problems in the psychotherapy of children with histories of incest." *American Journal of Psychotherapy* 34(1): 81–88.

Lamott, A. (1994). *Bird by Bird: Some Instructions on Writing and Life*. New York: Anchor Books.

Landis, C. (1940). *Sex in Development*. New York: Hoeber.

Landis, J. T. (1956). "Experiences of 500 children with adult sexual deviation." *Psychiatric Quarterly Supplement* 30(Part 1): 91–109.

Langer, E. J. (1975). "The illusion of control." *Journal of Personality and Social Psychology* 32: 311–328.

Langevin, R. (1990). "Sexual anomalies and the brain." In W. L. Marshall, D. R. Laws, and H. E. Barbaree, *Handbook of Sexual Assault: Issues, Theories, and Treatment of the Offender*. New York: Plenum Press. 103–113.

Lanyon, R. I. (1986). "Theory and treatment in child molestation." *Journal of Consulting and Clinical Psychology* 54(2): 176–182.

Lerner, M. J. (1980). *The Belief in a Just World: A Fundamental Delusion*. New York: Plenum Press.

Levine, J. (2002a). *Harmful to Minors*. Minneapolis: University of Minnesota Press.

Levine, J. (2002b, April 25). Letter to the editor. *Washington Times*.

Lewicki, P. (1984). "Self-schema and social information processing." *Journal of Personality and Social Psychology* 48: 463–574.

Lukianowicz, N. (1972). "Incest I: Paternal incest." *British Journal of Psychiatry* 120: 301–313.

Lustig, N., et al. (1966). "Incest: A family group survival pattern." *Archives of General Psychiatry* 14: 31–40.

Lykken, D. T. (1995). *The Antisocial Personalities*. Hillsdale, N.J.: Lawrence Erlbaum.

MacVicar, K. (1979). "Psychotherapeutic issues in the treatment of sexually abused girls." *Journal of the American Academy of Child Psychiatry* 18: 342–353.

Marks, G. (1984). "Thinking one's abilities are unique and one's opinions are common." *Personality and Social Psychological Bulletin* 10: 203–208.

Masson, J. (1984). *The Assault on Truth: Freud's Suppression of the Seduction Theory*. New York: Penguin Books.

Mathews, R., et al. (1989). *Female Sexual Offenders: An Exploratory Study*. Orwell, Vt.: Safer Society Press.

Matlin, M. W., and D. Stang (1978). *The Pollyanna Principle: Selectivity in Language, Memory, and Thought*. Cambridge, Mass.: Schenkman.

Michaud, S. G. (1994). *Lethal Shadow*. New York; Penguin Books.

Michaud, S. G., and H. Aynesworth (1989). *Ted Bundy: Conversations with a Killer*. New York: Penguin Books.

Miller, G., and S. Tompkins (1977). *Kidnapped! At Chowchilla*. Plainfield, N.J.: Logos International.

Mirkin, H. (1999). "The pattern of sexual politics: Feminism, homosexuality and pedophilia." *Journal of Homosexuality* 37: 2.

Mohr, J. W., et al. (1964). *Pedophilia and Exhibitionism*. Toronto: University of Toronto Press.

Motiuk, L. L., and S. L. Brown (1996). "Factors related to recidivism among released federal sex offenders." Presented at the XXVI International Congress of Psychology, Montreal, Canada.

Mrazek, D. (1985). "Science, politics, and ethics: Issues in the study of the sexual use of children." *Contemporary Psychology* 30(1): 37–38.

Mullen, P. E., et al. (1993). "Childhood sexual abuse and mental health in adult life." *British Journal of Psychiatry* 163: 721–732.

Nack, W., and D. Yaeger (1999, September 13). "Every Parent's Nightmare." *Sports Illustrated*.

National Campaign to Prevent Teen Pregnancy (2000). "Not Just Another Thing to Do: Teens Talk About Sex, Regret and the Influence of Parents." Washington, D.C.: National Campaign to Prevent Teen Pregnancy.

Nelson, E. C., et al. (2002). "Association between self-reported childhood sexual abuse and adverse psychosocial outcomes. Results from a twin study." *Archives of General Psychiatry* 59(2): 139–145.

Neuman, D. A., et al. (1996). "The long-term sequelae of childhood sexual abuse in women: A meta-analytic review." *Child Maltreatment* 1: 6–16.

Nichols, H. R., and I. Molinder (1996). *Multiphasic Sex Inventory II Handbook*. Tacoma, Wash.: Nichols & Molinder Assessments.

Nickerson, C. A. E., and K. R. Hammond (1993). "Comment on Ekman and O'-Sullivan." *American Psychologist* 48: 989.

Norris, F. H. (1992). "Epidemiology of trauma: frequency and impact of different potentially traumatic events on different demographic groups." *Journal of Consulting and Clinical Psychology* 60(3): 409–418.

Oddone, E., and M. L. Genuis (1996). *A Meta-Analysis of the Published Research on the Effects of Child Sexual Abuse*. Calgary, Canada: National Foundation for Family Research and Education.

Ondersma, S. J., et al. (2001). "Sex with children is abuse: Comment on Rind, Tromovitch, and Bauserman (1998)." *Psychological Bulletin* 127(6): 707–714.

Paolucci, E. O., et al. (2001). "A meta-analysis of the published research on the effects of child sexual abuse." *Journal of Psychology* 135(1): 17–36.

Paulhus, D. L. (1998). "Interpersonal and intrapsychic adaptiveness of trait self-enhancement: A mixed blessing." *Journal of Personality and Social Psychology* 74: 1197–1208.

Phillips, L. M. (1999). "Recasting consent: Agency and victimization in adult-teen relationships." In S. Lamb, *New Versions of Victims: Feminists Struggle with the Concept.* New York: New York University Press.

Plutarch (1992). *Plutarch's Lives.* New York: Random House.

Pope, K. S., and B. G. Tabachnick (1995). "Recovered memories of abuse among therapy patients: A national survey." *Ethics & Behavior* 5(3): 237–248.

Prentky, R. A., et al. (1997). "Recidivism rates among child molesters and rapists: A methodological analysis." *Law & Human Behavior* 21(6): 635–659.

Rascovsky, M., and A. Rascovsky (1950). "On consummated incest." *Journal of Psychoanalysis* 31: 42–47.

Reed, G. M., et al. (1994). "'Realistic acceptance' as a predictor of decreased survival time in gay men with AIDS." *Health Psychology* 13: 299–307.

_____ (1999). "Negative HIV-specific expectancies and AIDS-relate bereavement as predictors of symptom onset in asymptomatic HIV-positive gay men." *Health Psychology* 18: 354–363.

Regan, R. T. (1971). "Effects of a favor and liking on compliance." *Journal of Experimental Social Psychology* 7: 627–639.

Revitch, E., and R. G. Weiss (1962). "The pedophiliac offender." *Diseases of the Nervous System* 23: 73–78.

Rezendes, M., and M. Carroll (2002, April 8). "Boston diocese gave letter of assurance about Shanley: Told Calif. parish record was clean." *Boston Globe.*

Rind, B. (1995). "First do no harm: The sexual abuse industry." *Paidika: The Journal of Paedophilia* 3(12): 79–83.

Rind, B., et al. (1998a). "A meta-analytic examination of assumed properties of child sexual abuse using college samples." *Psychological Bulletin* 124: 22–53.

_____ (1998b). "An examination of assumed properties of child sexual abuse based on nonclinical samples." Paper presented at the symposium The Other Side of the Coin, sponsored by the Foundation for Church Work, Rotterdam, The Netherlands.

_____ (1999, November 6). "The clash of media, politics, and science: An examination of the controversy surrounding the *Psychological Bulletin* meta-analysis on assumed properties of child sexual abuse." Paper presented at the 1999 Joint Annual meeting of the Society for the Scientific Study of Sexuality and American Association of Sex Educators, Counselors and Therapists, St. Louis, Mo.

_____ (2000). "Science versus orthodoxy: Anatomy of the congressional condemnation of a scientific article and reflections on remedies for future ideological attacks." *Applied and Preventive Psychology* 9: 211–225.

_____ (2001a). "Moralistic psychiatry, Procrustes' bed, and the science of child sexual abuse: A reply to Spiegel." *Sexuality and Culture* 5: 75–85.

_____ (2001b). "The validity and appropriateness of methods, analyses and conclusions in Rind et al.: A rebuttal of victimological critique from Ondersma et al. (2001) and Dallam et al. (2002)." *Psychological Bulletin* 127(6): 734–758.

_____ (2001c, July/August). "The condemned meta-analysis on child sexual abuse: Good science and long-overdue skepticism." *Skeptical Inquirer* 25: 68–72.

Roesler, T. A., and T. W. Wind (1994). "Telling the secret: Adult women describe their disclosures of incest." *Journal of Interpersonal Violence* 9: 327–338.

Rosencrans, B. (1997). *The Last Secret*. Brandon, Vt.: Safe Society Press.

Rosenthal, R., and B. M. DePaulo (1979). "Sex differences in eavesdropping on nonverbal clues." *Journal of Personality and Social Psychology* 37: 273–285.

Rudacille, W. C. (1992). "Lies in disguise." *Text Analyst* 17.

_____ (1994). *Identifying Lies in Disguise*. Dubuque, Iowa: Kendall/Hunt Publishing.

Rush, F. (1980). *The Best Kept Secret: Sexual Abuse of Children*. New York: Mc-Graw-Hill.

Russell, D. E. H. (1984). *Sexual Exploitation: Rape, Child Sexual Abuse, and Workplace Harassment*. Newbury Park, Calif.: Sage.

Russell, D. H. (2000). *The Epidemic of Rape and Child Sexual Abuse in the United States*. Newbury Park, Calif.: Sage.

Salter, A. C. (1992). *Epidemiology of Child Sexual Abuse*. New York: Lawrence Erlbaum.

_____ (1995). *Transforming Trauma: A Guide to Understanding and Treating Adult Survivors of Child Sexual Abuse*. Newbury Park, Calif.: Sage.

Saradjian, J. (1996). *Women Who Sexually Abuse Children: From Research to Clinical Practice*. New York: John Wiley.

Saunders, B. (2001, October). "Family resolution therapy in cases of intrafamilial sexual abuse." Paper presented at the Midwest Conference on Child Sexual Abuse, Madison, Wisc.

Sauzier, M. (1980). "Disclosure of child sexual abuse: For better or for worse." *Psychiatric Clinics of North America* 12(2): 455–469.

Saywitz, K. J., et al. (1991). "Children's memories of a physical examination involving genital touch: Implications for reports of child sexual abuse." *Journal of Consulting and Clinical Psychology* 59: 5.

Scheflin, A. W., and D. Brown (1996). "Repressed memory or dissociative amnesia: What the science says." *The Journal of Psychiatry and Law* 24(2): 143–188.

Scheppele, K. L., and P. B. Bart (1983). "Through women's eyes: Defining danger in the wake of sexual assault." *Journal of Social Issues* 39(2): 63–80.

Schlessinger, L. (1999, March 23). *The Dr. Laura Show* [radio broadcast]. Los Angeles, Calif.: Premier Radio Networks.

Serin, R. C. (1996). "Violent recidivism in criminal psychopaths." *Law and Human Behavior* 20: 207–217.

Shedler, J., et al. (1993). "The illusion of mental health." *American Psychologist* 48: 1117–1131.

Sloane, P., and E. Karpinski (1942). "Effects of incest on the participants." *American Journal of Orthopsychiatry* 12: 666–673.

Slovenko, R. (1971). "Statutory rape." *Medical Aspects of Human Sexuality* 5: 155–167.

Smith, D. W., et al. (2000). "Delay in disclosure from childhood rape: Results from a national survey." *Child Abuse and Neglect: The International Journal* 24(2): 273–287.

Sorensen, T., and B. Snow (1991). "How children tell: The process of disclosure in child sexual abuse." *Child Welfare League of America* 70(1): 3–15.

Spiegel, D. (1990). "Trauma, dissociation, and hypnosis." In R. P. Kluft, *Incest Related Syndromes of Adult Psychopathology.* Washington, D.C.: American Psychiatric Press. 247–261.

"Statement of purpose." (1987). *Paidika: The Journal of Paedophilia* 1(1): 1–2.

Stein, J. A., et al. (1988). "Long-term psychological sequelae of child sexual abuse: The Los Angeles Epidemiologic Catchment Area Study." In G. E. Wyatt and G. J. Powell, *Lasting Effects of Child Sexual Abuse.* Newbury Park, Calif.: Sage. 135–154.

Steller, M., and G. Koehnken (1990). "Criteria based statement analysis." In D. C. Raskin, *Psychological Methods in Criminal Investigation and Evidence.* Portland, Oreg., Book News. 217–245.

Stevens, W. (1982). *The Collected Poems of Wallace Stevens.* New York: Vintage Books.

Swanson, D. W. (1968). "Adult sexual abuse of children." *Diseases of the Nervous System* 29(10): 677–683.

Taylor, S. E. (1989). *Positive Illusions: Creative Self-Deceptions and the Healthy Mind.* New York: Basic Books.

Taylor, S. E., and P. M. Gollwizer (1993). "The effect of mindset on positive illusions." *Journal of Personality and Social Psychology* 69: 213–226.

———— (1998). "Positive illusions." In H. Friedman, *Encyclopedia of Mental Health.* San Diego: Academic Press.

Taylor, S. E., and J. D. Brown (1988). "Illusion and well-being: A social-psychological perspective on mental health." *Psychological Bulletin* 103: 193–210.

Taylor, S. E., et al. (2000). "Psychological resources, positive illusions, and health." *American Psychologist* 55: 99–109.

Taylor, S. E., et al. (Submitted for publication). "Portrait of the self-enhancer: Well-adjusted, healthy, and appreciated by others, or maladjusted, unhealthy, and friendless."

Terman, L. (1951). "Correlates of orgasm adequacy in a group of 556 wives." *Journal of Psychology* 32: 115–172.

Terman, L. M. (1938). *Psychological Factors in Marital Happiness.* New York: McGraw-Hill.

Terr, L. (1990). *Too Scared to Cry.* New York: Harper and Row.

———— (1994). *Unchained Memories: True Stories of Traumatic Memories, Lost and Found.* New York: Basic Books.

Terr, L. C. (1985a). "Children traumatized in small groups." In S. Eth and R. S. Pynoos, *Post-Traumatic Stress Disorder in Children.* Washington, D.C.: American Psychiatric Press. 47–70.

———— (1985b). "Psychic trauma in children and adolescents." *Psychiatric Clinics of North America* 8(4): 815–835.

Thornburgh, D., and H. S. Lin, eds. (in press). *Youth, Pornography, and the Internet*. Washington, D.C.: National Academy Press.

Tian, Y., et al. (2000). "Recognizing lower face action units for facial expression." *Proceedings of the 4th IEEE International Conference on Automatic Face and Gesture Recognition*, Grenoble, France.

_____ (2001). "Recognizing action units for facial expression analysis." *Transactions on Pattern Analysis and Machine Intelligence* 23(2): 97–115.

Tiger, L. (1979). *Optimism: The Biology of Hope*. New York: Simon & Schuster.

Timnick, L. (1985a, August 25). "22% in survey were child abuse victims." *Los Angeles Times*.

_____ (1985b, August 26). "Children's abuse reports reliable, most believe." *Los Angeles Times*.

Tjaden, P., and N. Thoennes (1998). "Prevalence, incidence, and consequences of violence against women: Findings from the National Violence Against Women Survey, National Institute of Justice." In U.S. Department of Justice, *Centers for Disease Control and Prevention: Research in Brief*.

Tormes, Y. (1968). *Child Victims of Incest*. Denver, American Humane Society: Children's Division.

Trepper, T. S., and M. J. Barrett (1989). *Systemic Treatment of Incest*. New York: Brunner/Mazel.

Underwager, R., and H. Wakefield (1993). "Interview with Ralph Underwager and Holida Wakefield." *Paidika: The Journal of Paedophilia* 3(1): 3–12.

Undeutsch, I. (1989). "The development of statement reality analysis." In J. C. Yuille, *Credibility Assessment*. Dordrecht, The Netherlands: Kluwer Academic. 101–120.

van der Kolk, B. A., et al., eds. (1996). *Traumatic Stress*. New York, Guilford Press.

Virkunnen, M. (1975). "Victim-precipitated pedophilia offenses." *British Journal of Criminology* 15(2): 175–180.

Warren, J. I., et al. (1996). "The sexually sadistic serial killer." *Journal of Forensic Sciences* 6: 970–974.

Wegner, D. M., et al. (1994). "The allure of secret relationships." *Journal of Personality and Social Psychology* 66(2): 287–300.

Weiner, I. B. (1962). "Father-daughter incest: A clinical report." *Psychiatric Quarterly* 36(1): 607–632.

Weinrott, M. R., and M. Saylor (1991). "Self-report of crimes committed by sex offenders." *Journal of Interpersonal Violence* 6(3): 286–300.

Weiss, J., E. Rogers, et al. (1955). "A study of girl sex victims." *Psychiatric Quarterly* 29: 1–27.

"When politics clashes with science: An examination of the controversy surrounding the *Psychological Bulletin* article meta-analysis on the assumed properties of child sexual abuse." (2000). Flyer for symposium lead by Bruce Rind and Carol Tavris. Knoxville, Tenn.

Williams, L. M. (1992). "Adult memories of childhood abuse: Preliminary findings from a longitudinal study." *The Advisor* 5: 19–20.

_____ (1994). "Recall of childhood trauma: A prospective study of women's memories of child sexual abuse." *Journal of Consulting and Clinical Psychology* 62: 1167–1176.

_____ (1995). "Recovered memories of abuse in women with documented child sexual victimization histories." *Journal of Traumatic Stress* 8: 649–673.

Wyatt, G. E., and G. J. Powell, eds. (1988). *Lasting Effects of Child Sexual Abuse.* Newbury Park, Calif.: Sage.

Yorukoglu, A., and J. P. Kemph (1966). "Children not severely damaged by incest with a parent." *Journal of the American Academy of Child Psychiatry* 5(1): 111–124.

Zuckerman, M., et al. (1981). "Verbal and nonverbal communication of deception." In L. Berkowitz, *Advances in Experimental Social Psychology.* San Diego: Academic Press. 1–59.

INDEX

Index

Index

Index